PLACENTA WIT

Funded by the Government of Canada
Financé par la gouvernement du Canada 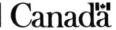 Canada

Demeter Press
140 Holland Street West
P. O. Box 13022
Bradford, ON L3Z 2Y5
Tel: (905) 775-9089
Email: info@demeterpress.org
Website: www.demeterpress.org

Demeter Press logo based on the sculpture "Demeter" by Maria-Luise Bodirsky
www.keramik-atelier.bodirsky.de

Printed and Bound in Canada

Front cover artwork: Jodi Selander, "Celestial Node," 2016, photograph and digital watercolor, 8x10. PlacentaLove.com

Library and Archives Canada Cataloguing in Publication

      Placenta wit : mother stories, rituals, and research / edited by Nané Jordan.

Includes bibliographical references.
ISBN 978-1-77258-107-2 (softcover)

      1. Birth customs. 2. Placenta. 3. Mothers. I. Jordan, Nané, 1968-, editor

GT2460.P63 2017   392.1'2   C2017-902498-1

PLACENTA WIT
Mother Stories, Rituals, and Research

EDITED BY
Nané Jordan

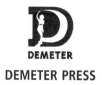

DEMETER

DEMETER PRESS

For my daughters,
Blessed be.

Table of Contents

Acknowledgements

This book is born from the genesis of my thirty-five years of involvement in midwifery and homebirth in Canada—and meeting many placentas over this time. It is to the placenta itself that I owe my gratitude of wonder. I have been a student, practitioner, doula, and researcher in the movement for more humane, woman- and mother-centred birth practices. I am, thus, indebted to, and grateful for, all the midwives, mothers, babies, and placentas, past and present, with whom I have worked and met over these years, as well as the wonderful proliferation of doulas into the birth scene in Canada. We need so much to acknowledge and honour each other and the various forms of labour we do throughout the many spheres and locations of birth giving, as well as the efforts of families to create a better and more loving world for their children from birth onwards.

I especially thank all the authors in this volume for your brilliant contributions. You inspire me. I so appreciate our shared enthusiasm for placentas and the community we made in the writing. Some authors, such as Janet Chawla, Polly Wood, Barbara Alice Mann, Farah Shroff, and Molly Remer, I thank for having already been colleagues on the placenta path.

I wish to acknowledge and thank my recent Social Sciences and Humanities Research Council of Canada postdoctoral tenure from 2014 to 2016 at the Centre d'Études Féminines et d'Études de Genre, at the University of Paris 8, France. This women and gender studies centre was inaugurated in 1974 by feminist writer-thinker Hélène Cixous, with whom, and with whose writing, I had the pleasure of deepening my thinking and practice of "birth"—birth as a way of living and writing. Without this period of research time and funding, and the treasure of my verdant Paris location and wanderings—actual, literary, and philosophic—this anthology, which gathers the gifts of many voices, would not have come to be. Thanks to Marie-Dominique Garnier in this regard and Anne E. Berger for appreciating my red thread ways and for supporting me to keep doing my feminist scholarship "otherwise."

This book has come at a key time in my life, at mid-life—and is a culmination of many pathways of being a daughter, sister, partner, mother, friend, midwife, doula, artist, scholar and researcher, community worker, traveller, and devotee of birth and the sacred female/feminine. I thank my stepmom, Faye, and my dad, Eric, for your love and encouragement, and for Evan's homebirth, so long ago attended by Mary, the lovely midwife with the long braids and soft voice. I give thanks for and to my sister Adia, a dear sister and friend and my cheering section.

My involvement in not only birth communities but in innovative and alternate women's scholarly circles has nourished me to do the creative work and woman-centred research that I yearned to do. In 2001, I found what I was looking for in the Women's Spirituality MA program, formerly based out of New College of California in San Francisco. My gratitude goes to mentors—Vicki Noble, Dianne Jenett, and Judy Grahn—and to alumna and dear friends in these circles of study and to others I met along the goddess way. Here was and is the power of following your heart, daydreaming, long conversations, and time spent with others in the struggles and joys of birthing a more just, sacred, and sustainable world. Onwards into Canadian academe, I thank my arts-based educational research colleagues, who encouraged my waxing poetic on placentas and trees, especially, life writers Erika Hasebe-Ludt and Carl Leggo, and philosopher Daniel Vokey. I also especially thank Gestare, my women's art collective, with whom so many streams of my life converge, in all we do to gestate womb space for art making and life. Thank you Barbara, Medwyn, and others from our collective over the years.

In 2002, I gave my first academic presentation at an Association for Research on Mothering conference in Toronto on the topic of my master's level homebirth research. My pathway with placentas was especially nourished in this scholarly venue of motherhood studies with ARM, now MIRCI, and Demeter Press itself—whose many books and authors I love to read and always relish, whose wise words carry me forward. What a pleasure and gift to contribute this volume to the chorus! I count the amazing MIRCI and Gift Economy conference in Rome, Italy, 2015, attended with Barbara Bickel and Vicki Noble, as the midwifery I needed for this book. Thank you to Andrea O'Reilly for all you do and for your encouragement in Rome to produce this volume—a timely undertaking. With continuing thanks to all at Demeter Press, to Angie for keeping me posted and organized, and to Jesse for your editing insight and care.

I also want to acknowledge philosopher Genevieve Vaughan, who opened my thinking toward the maternal gift economy, from which I deepened the roots for placental thinking. Gen saw the gifting relations of the placenta in my presentation at the ARM and Gift Economy conference in Toronto in 2008 and invited me to Rome to share more—grazie! Thus, like the many nourishing networks of vascular placental roots, it is my evolvement and exchange within richly interconnecting communities and relations that my vision, voice, and creative work is gestated and born. Not least in this nourishing network, I thank my family—Chris, Danaan, and Shanti—for all our birthings and your love and for laughing at your mama who types so very loudly on her old keyboard. I love you all the more.

Introduction

NANÉ JORDAN

MY FAVOURITE PLACENTA METAPHOR is that of a tree. The placenta, with its circular mass of vascular networks, resembles tree roots, interlacing as they extend into the nourishing soil of the earth. The umbilical cord is like a long tree trunk that grows up from these roots. Babies are the fruits and flowers on this human tree of life. A deeply symmetrical relationship exists between placentas and trees, as if we ritualize through our bodies the interconnections among living forms. And isn't there something radical about placentas? "Radical," as in the etymology of this word, which means "going to the roots." Placentas are radical, red, and bloody raw—the very rooty material of our maternal origins. After conception, placentas nourish our primary tie to life through a physical and symbolic relationship with our mothers. The placenta communicates this relationship through a dialogue of blood in pulsations of mother-baby heartbeats. Later, this placental language releases to the rhythms of birth. Secondary gifts of the placenta are then possible *after birth*.

Placenta Wit creatively and provocatively explores the placenta in mothers' contemporary and traditional uses of the human afterbirth. The word "wit" refers to intelligence and understanding, and knowledge gained. I like to think of "placenta wit" as the wisdom gathered over time by mothers and others, and from direct experiences of giving birth and mothering. Placenta interest and use is emerging in mothering and birth-care circles and discourses in North American and elsewhere. Some mothers are choosing to keep, bury, make art with, ceremonialize, or consume the placenta

1

after birth. My editorial intention was to gather an interdisciplinary range of placenta stories, rituals, and research, based on mothers' experiences, mother-centred practices, and emergent academic interest in this subject, in contemporary Canadian and American contexts but also beyond. This resulting volume highlights diverse understandings of the placenta, and its role in mothers' creative life giving. Authors explore homebirth, hospital-birth, midwifery, doula, feminist, and Indigenous perspectives. Through philosophical, literary, historical, poetic, legal, and economic analysis, the chapters depict the placenta's hidden role in the maternal meaning of life.

As such, this collection differs from scientific tomes on placenta pathology and evolution as well as midwifery volumes that forward the practical, therapeutic, and folkloric aspects of placentas (Ennings; Lim).[1] In contrast, *Placenta Wit* is not a how-to volume, nor does this anthology seek to promote one practice over another. The reader is advised to study widely and to consult with care providers if interested in placenta use. My hope is that *Placenta Wit* will contribute to a wider understanding of placentas, particularly an appreciation for and a valuing of the maternal roots of life, and the importance of and care for new mothers, who themselves care for new others in society at large.

As I write this introduction, I am also aware of mothers who would not have an interest in keeping their babies' placentas. The intention of this collection is not to forward any mandate on placenta use or nonuse but to hold space for mother-centred inquiry into this phenomena. I would note placenta use as a form of creative and/or reclaimed birth knowledge that can empower mothers and contribute to wellbeing. My own experiences with placentas emerged from pre-regulation Canadian midwifery and from mother-led philosophies of birth and postpartum care. I learned from mothers with various interests in their babies' placentas, as in their desires to keep, bury, consume, ceremonialize, or pursue such practices as "lotus birth." In lotus birth, the baby, cord and placenta are kept intact after birth, until the cord naturally dries and falls away from the baby's belly button, so that the placenta is released. Across North America, the movement to claim and use placentas has spread throughout a range of birth experiences, choices, and cultures—from home and hospital births to birth centres and from vaginal births to Caesarean sections. Yet there are limitations to choice when, as noted by author Valerie Borek herein, mothers are not legally able to keep their babies' placentas in all places.

By way of handling placentas, many new practices are emerging alongside precolonial ones, as held by Indigenous mothers and midwives. In this volume, such older placenta wisdom is explored by Barbara Alice Mann, who looks at placenta practices across Turtle Island (aka North America), and by Janet Chawla, who conducts research with traditional birth attendants in India. Additional chapters and perspectives include authors from such countries as Canada, the United States, England, Italy, Australia, and Mexico. Yet not all placenta practices are covered herein, such as the aforementioned "lotus birth" (Lim). Thus, although there are many voices in this volume, many are missing. By way of notation on the use of language in this volume, I draw from author Jonelle Myers to note that the terms "woman," "women," and "mother" and related pronouns are used by authors throughout. The editor "respectfully recognizes that some people who give birth may identify with another gendered term" or with nongendered terms, such as birthing person or birth giver (see Myers this volume).

Additionally, there are no direct analysis of faith-based protocols and scripture for handling placentas from religious traditions, such as Islam, Judaism, or Christianity. Such traditions may instruct upon the handling of birth blood and placentas as well as new motherhood, thus informing mothers' experiences, choices, and stories of such. Further volumes could expand upon placenta stories and research in a local and global sense, taking into account confluences of religious and cultural practices as these inform, shape, express or limit the birth-giving and postpartum experience as well as mothers' capacities to flourish.

In medicalized systems of birth care, the placenta, considered to be a human blood product, is often viewed as medical waste and/or as the object of research but not as the mother's or baby's body and property. Globally, birth experiences differ widely in terms of access to medical care during pregnancy and birth. Despite arguments for more medical access for mothers worldwide in rich nations and poor, many contributors to this anthology are critical of the current medical system in regards to birth, and notions of placentas within such. Although mothers benefit from medical care and treatment in pregnancy and birth, the medicalization of birth has also contributed to controlling and limiting women's birth choices and experiences (Davis-Floyd, *American Rite*; van Teijlingen et al.). As noted by feminist analysis, in some cases, the rights and agency of women themselves have been devalued as they give birth—a systemic effect of historical and contemporary patriarchy, and the confluence of such with social and medical practices (Cixous; Daly; O'Brien). Across North America and beyond, medicalization may pose limitations to understanding the importance and positive benefits of mother-centred practices, including mothers' access to placentas after birth.

Even when medical interventions are necessary for mothers and babies, birth remains much more than a medical event. It is a holistic, social, cultural, familial, spiritual, and community arrival of one being from another, having great impact for mothers and all beings. Mothers may have limited options for accessing care-givers who can support woman-centred, physiological (the innate human capacity for giving birth, residing in the mother-baby duo), and culturally engaged birth care. In this sense, I believe we need mother-centred philosophies and practices of care in all places and levels of birth giving. Many people are working for the humane and socially just treatment of women and babies. Movements for birth justice and positive birth experiences seek respectful, adequate, and caring treatment of all mothers and babies in all places and ways of birth.[2] This includes addressing social inequalities based on race, class, gender and sexuality that can lead to negative birth outcomes and experiences. The World Health Organization now recognizes that every woman and birth giver has the "right to dignified, respectful care during pregnancy and childbirth."

Within this vein of critique and mother-centred activism, I hope to see the best of life-saving medical practices integrated with the best of physiological birth research, traditional birthing wisdom, woman-centred midwifery, and empathetic, respectful, relational, and positive birth care on all sides of practice. This integration may, in some places, be coming around. But there is much work to do to ensure social justice in birth as well as to safeguard the health, safety, and wellbeing of all mothers and babies. What does it look like to activate mother-centred birth practices in all places of birth? Authors in this volume answer this question with attention to the humble placenta itself. The placenta's use and value for mothers and babies is born upon the grounds of the physical, social, philosophical, emotional, spiritual, and political heart of mothers' birth experiences, needs, choices, and care.

HOMEBIRTH MIDWIFERY AND PLACENTAS

My working background in pre-regulation Canadian midwifery—as a student, doula, advocate, and woman-centred birth activist—informs what I have come to know and love about placentas. My studies in the 1990s were marked by the "a-legal" status of midwifery and homebirth in Canada. I attended homebirths with midwives in both Ontario and British Columbia. There were no accredited programs for formal midwifery study, and enacted barricades that supported doctors' primary medical authority, rather than midwives' care, for women giving birth in Canada. Midwifery was often viewed with suspicion yet was claimed and loved by those who had experience of it. Midwifery and homebirth practices had been reemerging in North America from the 1970s onwards. The natural birth movement was closely related to the women's movement and counterculture communities of the 1970s (Gaskin; Koehler; Parvati-Baker). Midwifery was (and is) a form of women's health activism that empowered mothers and their birth experiences and challenged what had become, through overuse of technology and medical interventions, a highly controlled and paternalistic hospital birth environment (Arms; Davis-Floyd, *American Rite*). As midwifery was reviving, historical community roots of midwifery and home-birthing traditions also came into view, including the work of the Grand midwives of African American communities (Charles Smith) and the birthing traditions and practices of Indigenous midwives in Canada (Simpson; National Aboriginal Council of Canada).

Through the concerted efforts of many, we now have professional midwives working in many Canadian provinces yet not in all places or for all women (Bourgeault et al.; Shroff). In my early birth writing, I would tire of spilling ink to justify the field by citing studies of the safety and efficacy of midwifery and home-birth (Johnson and Daviss). Midwifery tends toward low rates of intervention, and mothers report high satisfaction in regards to their birth experiences. My own reading and research have largely focused on birth stories as told by mothers and midwives, my fa-vourite "genre" (e.g., Young). Stories can transmit rich narratives and varied details of personal and social birth-giving experiences, embedded as these are in mothers' everyday lives, families, birth politics and immediate circumstances. I believe that such stories are at the heart of transforming the social paradigm of birth toward mother-centred philosophies and care.

I write all this to provide some context for how placentas made themselves known in my life. What makes this topic striking to me is how far placentas have come since my early years of homebirth study. Attending to placentas was an outgrowth of the holistic midwifery I was learning from. Mothers, babies, and families were situated at the centre of this care. Birth was understood to be a normal and natural life event, albeit an overwhelming, powerful, potentially fulfilling and even ecstatic one. At home, healthy mothers could give birth with little or no medical inter-ventions, surrounded by their loved ones and the knowledgeable and compassionate care of midwives. Unlike in the hospital, af-ter giving birth mothers had easy and continuing access to their babies' placentas. After examination of the placenta for health and completeness, the midwives I studied with took time to show a mother her baby's placenta and described the wonders of this amazing organ to her. Some mothers wanted to keep the placenta, often burying it, whereas others asked the midwives to dispose of it. There were also "placenta prints" to make by pressing each side of the placenta on white sheets of paper to create birth mementos of this round, rooted form and cord.

Beyond this, some midwives supported mothers to consume the placenta after birth, if they so chose. This practice was understood to provide vital energy, to speed recovery, and to ward off the baby blues. Yet this seemed to be the most radical of practices. The topic of eating placenta was and is shocking or amazing to many people. Certainly not all lay midwives were aware of or supported placenta consumption. On this point, it would be interesting to trace where and how this practice came back into contemporary midwifery. There is evidence for its historical use by mothers in Europe (Enning), as well as Chinese medicinal preparations of such. Consumption requires various methods of preparation and must be done in a timely way. Many other mammals consume this nourishing postbirth meal.

After the homebirth of my first baby, and despite helping other mothers to prepare theirs, I did not want to consume placenta myself. I had used a sterile method of candle cauterization to sever my daughter's cord from her placenta in the quiet hours after her birth, long after her cord had stopped pulsing, thus not cutting quickly with metal. As my daughter rested peacefully in my arms, we sang blessing songs until her cord separation was complete. This practice came from an experienced elder midwife and was thought to be gentle for the baby. I do not hear anything about this practice now, but it is interesting in hindsight. I then buried my daughter's placenta a few months later under a tree in the backyard of our rental house. My husband and I had pondered the best place for her placenta's burial, and our East Vancouver yard represented the place and energy of our daughter's arrival in our lives.

By the time I gave birth to my second daughter, I was firmly interested in placenta consumption. Upon returning home from my hospital birth and postpartum hemorrhage, I ate a little bit of placenta each day in the week after her birth. It was cooked and stored for me by a friend. I believe this contributed to my emotional and physical recovery, which took several weeks after a difficult birth. A humorous aftereffect of this was keeping the rest of my daughter's placenta in the freezer for many months—years in fact. We finally decided the location for its proper burial when she was three years old. Such a delay can be an unintended result of mothers keeping their placentas—what I would call the "freezer story." Many placentas await use in home freezers. Even with the best of intentions, mothers are preoccupied in the early days of caring for newborns. Placenta consumption, therefore, involves timely use and preparations, as do other rituals. Just as mothers need support and care in the weeks following giving birth, they often require help for placenta use from knowledgeable friends, midwives, doulas, grandmothers, or partners.

These kinds of practices thus differ from contemporary medicalized childbirth, in which mothers do not have access to their babies' placentas, nor can they intimately handle and use them. Yet through current midwifery and obstetrical medical movements that promote physiologically based birth care (Gaskin; Buckley; Leboyer; Odent; Yoshimura), deeper understandings of how to care for the placenta and cord during and after birth are coming forward. This complex and situated topic of mother-centred birthing practices deserves continued inquiry and research. Claiming and honouring the placenta may play a vital role in understanding the sacredness of birth and the gift of life that mothers bring.

PLACENTERRE

As you may have guessed, I am a midwifery and doula advocate. Research confirms that midwifery is a birth model that works and that doulas can offer support, comfort, and advocacy to mothers in all places of birth (Davis-Floyd, *Birth Models*; Castaneda and Johnson Searcy). Midwives and doulas support mothers' physical, emotional, mental, spiritual, and psychosocial wellbeing within diverse communities. My own thinking explores how midwifery, in philosophy and practice, can be a basis for transformative, social philosophies of birth and can contribute to mother-empowering community development (Jordan, "To Be a Midwife"). In my years of educating about mother-centred birth practices, I found that reconnecting people to placentas holds a compelling thread in regards to birth experience (Jordan, "A Poetics"). The idea of placenta and cord design can strike a primal, symbolic "cord," one in which we return to our maternal roots at the portal of our lives.

Thus, beyond all this placenta-usefulness jazz is the simple wonder and awe I feel toward the placenta for being just what it is—a vital organ at the roots of life. I am what author Molly Remer identifies in this volume as "an acolyte of birth." I feel mystical wonder in the courageous presence of birthing mothers and the newly born, as surely many others feel. I feel this wonder in the presence of placentas—in their organic, gifting designs of human, birth-given origins. The round, flat-bread shape of a placenta includes both a mother's and baby's side. The mother's side looks almost brainlike, with intersecting lobes as if it has a mind of its own. The baby's side holds the umbilical cord, which splays into rooted networks of blood vessels. Capillaries diffuse nutrients and oxygen to the baby from the mother, exchanging beneficial substances, while taking away and filtering out many harmful ones. All the while, the separate vascular and circulatory systems of mother and baby are maintained. Thus, despite one human being growing inside another, each is unique yet bound to the other through this relational design. As I meditate upon and with this amazing morphology of relational life, I am driven to think with and through the placenta in a "poetics of the placenta."

Thus, from waxing poetic, I further introduce *Placenta Wit* as organized into three sections with chapters that weave stories, rituals, and research. The authors' stories and research are juxtaposed with one another, chapter by chapter, in order to resonate or contrast in various ways for the reader. I chose the terms "stories," "rituals," and "research" to be an overview of the ways that placentas come to the fore of mothers' birthing experiences, choices, and wisdom. This process is communicated in "stories," which includes mothers' and partners' birth and postpartum placenta stories while birthing, caring, and parenting in the early days, weeks, and months of life. "Ritual" refers to the many ways in which the placenta has ceremonial and/or therapeutic values after birth. Rituals can be practices of use that impart meaningful social, symbolic, and/or spiritual effects. By "research," I mean how we inquire into the anatomical, physiological, ceremonial, therapeutic, and symbolic uses and values of placentas, including scientific, social, historical, humanistic, symbolic, literary and poststructural studies. Research can offer evidence, provide conclusions, or make recommendations about placenta use in this regard. In many cases, all three terms combine in the authors' work, as story, ritual, and research come together in the birthing of these texts.

I have titled each of the three sections of *Placenta Wit* as Placenterre I, II, and III, after author Marie-Dominique Garnier's creation of this term. "Placenta," in its Greek and Latin origins, means a "flat cake," symbiotic to its shape and perhaps culinary history.

One also sees and hears the word "place." Thus, "placenterre" combines "placenta" with "place," and includes the French word for earth, "*terre*." This word roots us to our "*place en terre*," our place on earth. In her chapter, Garnier weaves a literary journey through lost languages of placentas and birth, revealing female and maternal origins in the writing of feminist author Hélène Cixous. Garnier offers the term "placenterre" in "an effort to unite the placenta and the terrestrial, in other words to reconstruct a path between 'earth' and 'birth.'" She mirrors the "nourishing element" that emerges in Cixous's writing that displaces the dominating language of the phallus and the logocentrism of Western discourse. Thus, we might consider the "placenterre" as a basis for reimagining mother-centric philosophies and more nourishing ways of engaging with birth and with life.

Indeed, the placenta has a vegetal form with its tree morphology. Its leaflike shape is beautifully captured in the cover art for this book, a photographic image of a placenta titled "Celestial Node" and created by Jodi Selander. The vegetal structure of the placenta calls to the very life force it provides. This force is connected to both earth and the Earth, to which we might return placentas respectfully, or even consume their nourishing, leaflike forms.

In the first of six chapters of Placenterre I, Jonelle Myers introduces us to the term "placentophagy." She outlines the careful preparations that led to her empowered experiences of birth and early mothering, which included consuming placenta in capsule form for her "fourth trimester"—the intensive early days and weeks of mothering. Myers acknowledges that not all women have access to what she was able to pursue. She wonders how such education and resources could be available for all mothers, and recommends more research in order to continue the social normalization of honouring the natural birthing process. In "Beyond the Birth Room," Amy Stenzel critiques the separation of mothers and babies from their placentas in Western medical practice, including disposing of placentas as the singular option. Stenzel examines why and how this nourishing organ has been missing from Western feminist thought. She points to the importance of honouring the placenta as a way to heal society, to revalue maternity and caring relationships, and to build healthy human communities from the start of life.

In "Slightly Inappropriate but Really Brilliant," Nicole Link-Troen tells her story of becoming a specialist doula who supports mothers through placenta encapsulation. Link-Troen came to her birth work after experiences with her mother's Caesarian sections. Seeking birthing alternatives for herself, Link-Troen also found some magic in placenta pills and made a brilliant career turn of her own. In the next chapter, "I'm Just Going to Give You the Injection for the Placenta," British midwife Alys Einion examines the culture of risk that has led to the use of oxytocin medications that speed delivery of the placenta, and the language used to direct women toward this practice in midwifery care. Einion asks how and if midwives can hold true to their own philosophies of woman-centred care.

In "Placental Waste," Barbara Alice Mann, of Ohio Bear Clan, cautions us about the grave social and environmental risks inherent in mishandling placentas and umbilical cords postbirth. Mann explores historical and contemporary practices and teachings of the matriarchal cultures of Indigenous peoples across Turtle Island. She directs the discourse back to matriarchal principles as a corrective to Euro-patriarchal and colonial studies of Indigenous peoples. She discusses the complementary female to male poles of these lived philosophies, and the Twinned Cosmos of Blood (Mother Earth) and Breath (Brother Sky) practices, in which "everything has consciousness and balancing duties of some kind."

In "Discourses of Love and Loss," Emily Burns notes how "the placenta is so rarely afforded the attention of social research." Burns provides accounts of mothers' uses of placentas from her study of homebirth narratives in Australia. She analyzes how mothers' alternative placenta rituals have become a "meaningful way for women to engage with their birth experiences ... and [how placenta rituals] represent a complex combination of love and loss."

A series of placenta artworks by Catherine Moeller and Jodi Selander completes this section. Moeller describes and depicts the burial of her daughter's placenta under a tree. Selander, a placenta encapsulation specialist, explores the magnificence of placentas through her photographic art. We, thus, take an artful pause and breathe into the next section of chapters.

Placenterre II is comprised of six chapters and opens with one by birth educator, artist, and priestess Molly Remer. In her chapter "A Medal for Birth," Remer playfully considers herself an "acolyte of birth," as she honours the blood-red stains left on her floor after giving birth. She continues with storied accounts of her four births, and the ways in which she and her family greeted not only each baby but each placenta earthside. Her artwork leads to the jeweled creation that is "A Medal for Birth." Then, with a poetic turn, Farah M. Shroff gives thanks to her sons' placentas for their life-nourishing ways in "Planting our Placentas." Shroff poetically relates her family ceremonies of placenta burials under trees, and the mixing of Parsi and Afrikan cultures in her family line as she artfully offers the vivid, red life force of the placenta back to the earth.

In "Circling the Red Tent," Alison Bastien writes storied vignettes from daily life, working with mothers, babies, and placentas as a midwife in Mexico. Bastien questions the commodification of placentas through encapsulation specialists. She teaches mothers to steam and dry placentas for themselves, and writes descriptively of red tents, blood mysteries, motherlines, and placenta days, engaging mothers to reclaim and re-story "ownership of their own miraculous creations."

Italian midwife Amyel Garnaoui contributes some of the latest scientific discoveries about placentas in her chapter "The Amazing Placenta." Garnaoui discusses the problems arising from clamping the umbilical cord too early, the wonders of imprinted genes, the mother-father genomic debate, and the evolutionary basis for mothers' consumption of placentas. With so much science supporting mother- and baby-centred physiological birth, and favouring placenta care and use, Garnaoui asks why these practices are not more fully encouraged.

In the next chapter, "Maternal Roots," I explore placenta practices and rituals from my learning experiences in pre-regulation Canadian midwifery. I carry this grassroots background into an analysis of relations between the placenta and the maternal gift economy, as theorized by philosopher Genevieve Vaughan. I suggest that the placenta's gift "morphology" has metaphoric and practical purposes that we can keep in mind for locating and developing more mother-centred birth views and worldviews.

The second artful pause includes artwork from "The Birth Project" by artist Amanda Greavette. Her paintings represent "the real and symbolic nature of birth as a holistic experience" and as profound events in women's lives. Then, through "The Placenta Project," I explore the possibilities of a placenta-nature interface in textile art installations in trees and water, at the waterline of Lake Ontario, the very shores of my "placenterre" (place of birth).

Placenterre III continues to weave stories, rituals, and research, as Polly Wood examines the relationship between placentas, the economy, and menstrual blood in "Bledsung of the Placenta." Wood explores poet Judy Grahn's metaformic understanding of the menstrual origins of culture and Marilyn Waring's economic recounting of mothers' unpaid work. Wood exposes the loss of placentas through their lack of perceived economic "value" and the devaluation of women's life-giving blood. In storying her artistic and placenta encapsulation birth work, Wood gifts us her "bledsung" and sings out the sacred power of women's blood.

In "A Placenta by Any Other Name," attorney-at-law and mother Valerie Borek shares entwined stories of her experiences with placentas—as an attorney, as a mother, and as a woman. Borek's story includes assisting another mother with legal intervention to retrieve her baby's placenta from an American hospital. Borek poses the question "who owns the placenta?" and examines how this "powerful organ" has been marginalized and contained by authoritarian institutions of medicine and the law. In becoming a mother herself, Borek writes of her resulting journey toward the divine feminine through her own life-giving female body and her son's placenta, revaluing these sacred forms.

Grandmother and birth researcher Janet Chawla, of the JEEVA Research Project in Northern India, relates in her chapter "The Baby's Life Is in the Placenta Only" stories of birth and placenta wisdom from the Indigenous birth work of dais, or midwives, who care for poor and rural mothers across India. Dias work in remote villages, often far from hospitals, where the integrity of the placenta and cord is sacrosanct and a means of maintaining the baby's life after birth. The dais' voices and practices represent ancient arts of the midwife, handed down over generations of maternal care.

In "Placenta Wit and Chick Lit," author Judy Battaglia explores feminism, homebirth, placentas, academe, and the meaning of birth in Kimberly Knutsen's first novel *The Lost Journals of Sylvia Plath*. Battaglia enquires into the novel's characters—two of which are doctoral candidates. The book's characters think, talk about, and experience birth and placentas, while navigating the complexities of life, love, friendship, family, and betrayal. *Placenta Wit* is then completed with the chapter "Snakes, Berries, and Bears," a father's story of placenta life by Chris Cordoni, who happens to be my husband. Cordoni tells the tale of the hospital birth of our second child and the planting at home of her placenta in the West Coast forest of our family cabin. This is a father's storied view of a challenging hospital birth, contrasted with, and ultimately healed by, the nurturing, earthy routines of our daily lives at home and in the forest.

To conclude my introduction to *Placenta Wit*, I return to the idea that there is indeed something radical about claiming, planting, consuming, thinking, writing, art making, and creating ceremonies with placentas. Radical, as in going to the roots of our lives to connect with and honour birth-based and bodied life, where placentas are the very interface of maternal life-gifting origins. We can create the "placenterre," where earth and birth are reunited and mothers and birth givers are valued. To "wit," this may be the intelligence and wisdom arising from the placenta itself and from the years of birth work and activism by mothers, midwives, doulas, birth workers, and others. In this way, mother-centred practices, social justice, and positive, empowering birth care summon us to uncover, understand, and confront the challenges and limitations mothers face, as well as the potential for mothers' empowerment, wellbeing, insight, and joy.

I am inspired by it all. My heart opens in this work like attending a mother giving birth, a witness to her courage and strength. The authors in this anthology do justice in the full sense of that word to the placenta. I call out my thanks to all, for your placental thinking and wisdom, for beholding the nourishing roots of motherhood and life itself.

ENDNOTES

[1]In regards to postpartum placenta consumption for mothers' recovery and wellbeing after birth, Jodi Selander of Placenta Benefits shares information about the benefits of placenta consumption, trains placenta encapsulation practitioners, and conducts research on placentophagy via the encapsulation method. For information see www.placentabenefits.com

[2]An example of such a group is Black Women Birthing Justice. This group addresses social justice in birth for women of colour, low-income women, immigrant families, queer and transfolk, and incarcerated women. For more information, see www.blackwomenbirthingjustice.org/birth-justice. In addition, I take the term "positive birth" from a group identifying themselves as the Positive Birth Movement. For more information on the idea of positive birth and its potential scope of practices see the "Manifesto" at www.positivebirthmovement.org/our-manifesto

WORKS CITED

Arms, Suzanne. *Immaculate Deception II: Myth, Magic & Birth*. Celestial Arts, 1996.

Bourgeault, Lynn et al., editors. *Reconceiving Midwifery*. McGill-Queen's University Press, 2004.

Buckley, Sarah. *Gentle Birth, Gentle Mothering*. One Moon Press, 2005.

Castaneda, Angela N. and Julie Johnson Searcy, editors. *Doulas and Intimate Labour: Boundaries, Bodies, and Birth*. Demeter Press, 2015.

Charles Smith, Margaret. *Listen to Me Good: The Story of an Alabama Midwife*. Ohio State University Press, 1996.

Cixous, Hélène. "Laugh of the Medusa." Translated by Keith Caplan and Paula Cohen. *Signs*, vol. 1, no. 4, 1976, pp. 875-893.

Daly, Mary. *Beyond God the Father: Towards a Philosophy of Women's Liberation*. Beacon Press, 1973.

Davis-Floyd, Robbie E. *Birth as an American Rite of Passage*. University of California Press, 1992.

Davis-Floyd, Robbie E. et al. *Birth Models that Work*. University of California Press, 2009.

Enning, Cornelia. *Placenta: Gift of Life. The Role of the Placenta in Different Cultures and How to Prepare and Use it as Medicine.* Motherbaby Press, 2007.

Gaskin, Ina May. *Spiritual Midwifery.* 3rd ed. The Book Publishing Company, 1990.

Gaskin, Ina May. *Birth Matters: A Midwife's Manifesto.* Seven Stories Press, 2011.

Johnson, Kenneth C., and Betty-Anne Daviss. "Outcomes of Planned Home Births with Certified Professional Midwives: Large Prospective Study in North America." *British Medical Journal,* vol. 330, no 1416, 2005, BMJ, doi: https://doi.org/10.1136/bmj.330.7505.1416.

Jordan, Nané. "A Poetics of the Placenta: Placental Cosmology as Gift and Sacred Economy." A (M)otherworld is Possible: Two Feminist Visions, The Association for Research On Mothering Annual Conference, 2009, York University, Toronto. Conference Presentation.

Jordan, Nané. "To Be a Midwife: Overcoming the Obstacles in Canada, Part 2." *The Practicing Midwife,* vol. 18, no. 8, 2015, pp. 30-32.

Koehler, Nan. *Artemis Speaks: V.B.A.C. Stories and Natural Childbirth Information.* Jerald R. Brown, 1985.

Leboyer, Frederick. *Birth without Violence.* Alfred A. Knopf, 1975.

Lim, Robin. *Placenta: The Forgotten Chakra.* Half Angel Press, 2010.

National Aboriginal Council of Canada (NACM). Aboriginal Midwifery in Canada, 2012, aboriginalmidwives.ca. Accessed 14 Nov. 2016.

O'Brien, Mary. *The Politics of Reproduction.* Routledge and Kegan, 1981.

Parvati Baker, Jeannine. *Prenatal Yoga & Natural Birth.* 1974. Freestone Publishing Company, 1986.

Selander, Jodi. "Placenta Benefits Info: Avoid the Baby Blues." *Placenta Benefits,* 2017, placentabenefits.info. Accessed 10 Oct. 2016.

Simpson, Leanne. "Birthing an Indigenous Resurgence: Decolonizing Our Pregnancy and Birthing Ceremonies." *"Until Our*

Hearts Are on the Ground": Aboriginal Mothering, Oppression, Resistance and Rebirth, edited by D. Memee Lavell-Harvard and Jeannette Corbiere Lavell, Demeter Press, 2006, pp. 25-33.

Shroff, Farah, editor. *The New Midwifery: Reflections on Renaissance and Regulation.* Women's Press, 1997.

van Teijlingen, E. et al., editors. *Midwifery and the Medicalization of Childbirth: Comparative Perspectives.* Nova Science Publishers, 2004.

World Health Organization (WHO). "Prevention and Elimination of Disrespect and Abuse During Childbirth." WHO, http://www.who.int/reproductivehealth/topics/maternal_perinatal/statement-childbirth/en/. Accessed 8 Apr. 2017.

Yoshimura, Tadashi. *Joyous Childbirth Changes the World.* Seven Stories Press, 2014.

Young, Catherine. *Mother's Best Secrets.* Mother Press, 1992.

PLACENTERRE I

1.
Placenta Consumption

Fourth-Trimester Energy Force and Source of Empowerment

JONELLE MYERS

THIS NARRATIVE FOCUSES ON THE EFFECT of placenta consumption, or placentophagy, on my breastfeeding, fourth-trimester, and return to work experience. I first set the foundation of my story by sharing my prenatal experience. Preparing for birthing my child was an empowering experience that set the tone for my mothering and overall positive outcomes in breastfeeding. My body was growing an entirely new human being inside my womb: the realization of the magnitude of continuing the human existence was powerful. My prenatal experience—in which I was accompanied by a supportive and loving husband/birth partner as well as compassionate and noninterventionist midwives of the local university birthing centre—was an exercise in accepting the natural, biologically normal process of pregnancy and breastfeeding. Claiming the birth experience as my own was also a feminist statement of liberation.

During my prenatal preparation, I learned of all my options of birthing: informed consent to pain relief and labour-hastening interventions; body positioning to facilitate an easy birthing experience; optimal golden hour processes; and placental consumption in raw and encapsulated forms. I attended a five-week Mongan Method hypnobirthing class, during which my husband and I learned about this practice and philosophy of birthing as well as how to advocate for our family, my body, and my baby in the event that the medical establishment applied pressure to intervene in my birthing experience. The knowledge I gained during this class as well as the camaraderie I developed with other likeminded mothers and partners contributed to my confidence as a first-time mother.[1] This powerful prenatal experience solidified my role as the mother and ensured my right to the birth that I wanted and deserved.

Similar to my birthing goals, I decided early during pregnancy that successful breastfeeding was not just a goal but the baseline of my experience. Breastfeeding is the biological norm and a source of empowerment to reclaim the infant feeding practice, which patriarchal capitalist biomedicine and advertising have historically demeaned and usurped (Stevens et al.; Parry et al.; Madden). I also knew that I had the support of my partner and midwife and, again, took a class to prepare myself for breast-feeding. This Breastfeeding 101 class, hosted by the university hospital and birth centre, was not covered by my insurance. I paid out of pocket and attended during my third trimester. I also attended a local breastfeeding support group, which was a moving experience. This was my first time surrounded by over two-dozen women who were nursing their children of various ages. Several International Board Certified Lactation Consultants (IBCLC) were available to answer questions. I attended with a long-time friend who had her third child just a month before I was expecting my son to emerge. The support of the local breastfeeding community and this dear friend were additional sources of support I accessed during the fourth trimester.

After completing the hypnobirthing and breastfeeding classes, I further researched placentophagy. Many online resources praised the benefits of placenta consumption, and the Birth Education Center of San Diego, where we attended the hypnobirthing class, provided a comprehensive list of those benefits:

- •can curb postpartum depression ("baby blues")
- •replenishes nutrients and is a natural painkiller
- •is shown to increase milk production
- •increases energy after birth, combats fatigue
- •is made perfectly for you, because it is you
- •helps stop or lessen postpartum bleeding after birth
- •provides natural iron supplementation after birth
- •helps with insomnia or sleep disorders
- •helps contract uterus back to normal size.

I decided to consume my placenta, in both raw and encapsulated forms, with the hope that I would experience the benefits touted by proponents. Truly believing and visualizing general positive outcomes of birthing and breastfeeding are practices of hypnobirthing (Mongan), and I applied them to placentophagy. I learned of the many benefits of placenta consumption, which, whether real or not, were real in their consequences (Thomas and Thomas qtd. in Ferris).

BIRTHING EXPERIENCE

My birthing experience was calm, gentle, and quick. My dear son was born after eight hours of peaceful labour. The only medical intervention I received was intravenous fluids for dehydration, approximately seven hours into labour. I did not have any medication, as I did not feel any pain, just pressure and mild discomfort. Another practice of hypnobirthing is to breathe into discomfort and to visualize the changes in the body. Surges (commonly known as contractions) are natural movements to be welcomed, much like co-meditation breathing in yoga (Farhi). I contribute these techniques to my overall pleasant birthing and recovery experience. The midwives and nurses attending my birth were all supportive of and knowledgeable about hypnobirthing, so as to facilitate my birth plan. They respected my desire for a nonmedicated, nonintervention birth.

My midwife and delivery team respected the golden hour: the critical time after the baby has birthed, in which mother and child interaction begins (Odent). My son was placed onto my chest, skin-to-skin, immediately after he emerged from my womb. During the golden hour, my husband and I simply enjoyed our son, gazing into his eyes, smelling his skin, basking in the joy of our new family. Although the golden hour is a time of serene bonding, many processes occurred in our birthing room. We delayed umbilical cord clamping and cutting to assist our son with a smooth transition to the world (Haelle). Our son crawled to my right breast, rooted, and latched to begin breastfeeding. During this precious time, an OB/GYN resident of the university labour and delivery department suggested to me that I receive artificial oxytocin to hasten the delivery of my placenta. My midwife reminded the OB/GYN resident of my birth plan and that I had requested no interventions, including the delivery of my placenta. We waited what seemed like just a few moments, which was likely twenty to thirty minutes, and my placenta emerged. I thank my midwife for asserting my request for a medication-free birthing experience while I was in the trance of the golden hour.

FOURTH TRIMESTER

Within hours, my placenta encapsulationist picked up my placenta from the birth centre, which my nurse had packaged neatly in a cooler with ice. Consuming the first raw portions of my placenta within twenty-four hours gave me the physical and mental boost to truly *believe* my breastfeeding relationship would be positive. My baby lost 10.3 percent of his birth weight at discharge, thirty-two hours postbirth—from 107 ounces to 96 ounces. This amount of weight loss is normal, especially for women who receive intravenous fluids during labour (Noel-Weiss et al). However, my midwives were slightly concerned and requested a weight check with our primary care physician the day after discharge. I kept my baby on my breast as much as possible, skin-to-skin, and continued to consume my raw placenta per the dosage recommended by my encapsulationist. His weight gradually increased at each appointment, and by seventeen days of age, he surpassed his birth weight while being exclusively breastfed.

My fourth-trimester experiences were overwhelmingly ideal. My breastfeeding relationship with my baby was healthy and successful. My mood was regulated, with no "baby blues." I was truly filled with warmth and enjoyment in my new role as mother. My body recovered quickly, and I was practising postpartum yoga and walking the family dog within weeks. I experienced only mild discomfort: from approximately four hours postpartum and throughout the fourth trimester, I sporadically consumed over-the-counter acetaminophen for mild aches and pains. All this time, I was consuming my raw and/or encapsulated placenta. I also found a loving breastfeeding support group that met after postpartum yoga, led by dually certified IBCLC yoga instructors.

RETURNING TO WORK

Preparing to return to work was an emotional experience. I had just spent the last twenty weeks with my brand new baby, almost every moment of every day. Our breastfeeding relationship was working well, and we had no challenges beyond the typical birth weight loss. From the time my baby was five weeks old, I had been pumping my breasts with a consumer-grade double electric breast pump provided by my health insurance. I pumped once every other day, enough to get my body acclimated to pumping—to learn a routine, build a freezer supply for times separated from baby, and create an emergency backup supply in case of unforeseen separation. While I was preparing my physical body, I also needed to prepare my mind. I knew I wanted to consume my placenta capsules as part of my preparation to return to work, so I saved approximately six weeks supply of capsules. Based on stories from other working mothers, I expected to experience anxiety when separated from my baby and also a decreased milk supply.

Thankfully, my baby was enrolled in the childcare centre located and operated by my employer. My office is three miles away from the childcare centre, and travel takes ten minutes. Having my baby so close and with my esteemed colleagues was relieving. But I knew I was at risk of emotional distress during those first few weeks of separation. I read about the potential heartbreak, the separation anxiety, and the worry women experience. A friend with a baby just two months older than mine shared her experience of tearful goodbyes at the morning drop off, emotional breakdowns in the car, and wistful days dreaming about pickup. I was determined to mitigate these negative feelings as much as possible. I had negotiated returning to work on a part-time basis, so my son would be in childcare three days per week.

To prepare my return, I again consumed my encapsulated placenta starting two weeks before my first day back in the office, at twenty weeks postpartum. Reintroducing my own perfect blend of hormones and energy, through ingesting the placenta, kept my emotions regulated; it was a natural mood stabilizer. In addition to placenta consumption, the week before my return to work, my baby and I spent about eight hours over three days in his classroom relaxing, playing, breastfeeding, getting to know the classroom space, and meeting his peers and teachers.

With dismal parental leave policies in the United States, I am thankful for the policies in California that supported my twenty-two weeks of job-protected leave, sixteen of which had partial wage replacement. On my first day back to work, my baby and I arrived at the childcare centre early, breastfed peacefully, and then I went to my office. Although I missed my son dearly, I acclimated back into the workforce easily, without emotional distress, and with sufficient breast pumping output. I needed ten to fifteen ounces of pumped breast milk for my baby each day. With three pumping sessions over nine hours of separation, I produced just that. At the time of this writing, nine months have passed since I've returned to work. I continue to pump breast milk three times per day for my son, and my daily average is approximately twelve ounces.

POSITIVE OUTCOMES

Were my positive fourth-trimester and return-to-work outcomes correlated with placenta encapsulation? Or was placenta encapsulation merely one of many factors contributing to my positive outcomes? Although I cannot know the direct effect of placenta consumption on my experience, I do contribute my positive outcomes at least partially to placentophagy. Placenta consumption was one of many factors contributing to my success, which cannot be discounted. In fact, all mothers should have access to affordable placenta encapsulating services, breastfeeding education and support groups, sufficiently paid family leave, supportive employers, part-time and flexible work schedules, and onsite or nearby childcare facilities.

In addition to the lived experience of an unmedicalized birth, exclusive breastfeeding and placentophagy, these acts resist the patriarchal medical hegemony of birthing and feeding babies. Historically, in the United States and elsewhere, women and babies have been alienated from the birthing experience in favour of doctor- and hospital-centred birth in the capitalist patriarchal economy (Cahill; Demanuele; Haire qtd. in Young). In recent years, women have reclaimed the birthing experience, and the medical establishment has begun to shift to women- and baby-centred birthing. The Baby Friendly Hospital Initiative has institutionalized many pro-breastfeeding policies, but only for hospitals that participate. We must continue the social normalization of honouring the natural birthing process and of understanding breastfeeding as the biological norm and the placenta as an energy source.

LIMITATIONS

Access to placentophagy must be widened to women of all socioeconomic and cultural backgrounds. My middle-class status provided access to services that may not be available to other women; these services may be cost prohibitive to other women. My prenatal hypnobirthing classes, breastfeeding classes and placenta encapsulation were not covered under my health insurance, and, therefore, I paid out-of-pocket. Affordable and accessible birth and breastfeeding classes, as well as placenta encapsulation, need to be expanded and covered by health insurance. Whether a true or placebo effect, this cost may prevent the need for more intervention into breastfeeding, such as lactation consultations, and also prevent the need to supplement breastfeeding with expensive artificial milk. Additional research into placentophagy is desperately needed to understand the full effect of this practice.

CONCLUSION

Placentophagy was one of several assets I drew upon to contribute to my positive and empowering birthing and breastfeeding experiences, from my child's birthday through the first year of life and to my returning to work and beyond. Although I cannot attribute my successful experience directly to consuming my placenta, I have accepted it as a meaningful part of my journey. Prenatal preparation via hypnobirthing and breastfeeding classes, respectful midwifery, the golden hour, breastfeeding support groups and IBCLC's, and supportive employers all contributed to my successful breastfeeding relationship with my baby. Claiming placentophagy, along with unmedicalized birth, as woman- and baby-centred practices places the entitlement to natural birthing in the lives of women and families. We must continue to work toward equal and affordable access to prenatal, birth, and fourth-trimester options for all women.

ENDNOTE

[1]The terms "woman," "women," "mother" and related pronouns have been used throughout this article. The writer respectfully makes recognition that some people who give birth may identify with another gender term.

WORKS CITED

Baby-Friendly USA, Inc. "Baby Friendly Hospital Initiative." *Baby Friendly USA*, 2012, https://www.babyfriendlyusa.org/. Accessed 29 Mar. 2016.

Birth Education Center of San Diego. "What is Encapsulation?" *The Birth Education Center of San Diego*, 2016, birtheducationcenter.com. Accessed 19 Jan. 2016.

Cahill, Heather A. "Male Appropriation and Medicalization of Childbirth: An Historical Analysis." *Journal of Advanced Nursing*, vol. 33, no.3, 2001, pp. 334-342. *Wiley Online Library*, doi: 10.1046/j.1365-2648.2001.01669. Accessed 24 May 2016.

Demanuele, Gaye. "Why Birth is a Feminist Issue." *The Freedom Socialist Organiser*, 2013, https://www.socialism.com/drupal-6.8/organiser-articles/why-birth-feminist-issue. Accessed 24 May 2016.

Farhi, Donna. *The Breathing Book: Good Health and Vitality Through Essential Breath Work*. Holt Publishing, 1996.

Ferris, Kerry. *The Real World*. W. W. Norton & Company, 2014.

Haelle, Tara. "Delayed Umbilical Cord Clamping May Benefit Children Years Later." *National Public Radio*, 26 May 2015, http://www.npr.org/sections/health-shots/2015/05/26/409697568/delayed-umbilical-cord-clamping-may-benefit-children-years-later. Accessed 29 Mar. 2016.

Madden, Caolan. "Breastfeeding and Capitalism: A Provocation." *Weird Sister*, 1 Sept. 2015, http://weird-sister.com/2015/09/01/breastfeeding-and-capitalism-a-provocation/. Accessed 24 May 2016.

Mongan, Marie. *HypnoBirthing: The Mongan Method: A Natural Approach to a Safe, Easier, More Comfortable Birthing.* Health Communications Inc., 2005.

Noel-Weiss, Joy, et al. "An Observational Study of Associations Among Maternal Fluids during Parturition, Neonatal Output, and Breastfed Newborn Weight Loss." *International Breastfeeding Journal,* vol. 6, no. 9, 2011, pp. 1-10. *NCBI,* doi: 10.1186/1746-4358-6-9. Accessed 24 May 2016.

Odent, Michael. "The First Hour Following Birth: Don't Wake the Mother!" *Midwifery Today: The Heart and Science of Birth,* vol. 61, 2002, pp. 9-11, https://www.midwiferytoday.com/articles/firsthour.asp. Accessed 24 May 2016.

Parry, Kathleen, et al. "Understanding Women's Interpretations of Infant Formula Advertising." *Birth Issues in Perinatal Care,* vol. 40, no. 2, 2013, pp.115-124. Wiley Library Online, doi: 10.1111/birt.12044. Accessed 17 May 2016.

Stevens, Emily, et al. "A History of Infant Feeding." *The Journal of Perinatal Education,* vol. 18, no. 2, 2009, pp. 32-39. *NCBI,* doi: 10.1624/105812409X426314. Accessed 29 Mar. 2016.

Young, Diony. "'It Is Better to Light One Candle than to Curse the Darkness': The Legacy of Doris Haire." *Birth Issues in Perinatal Care,* vol. 41, no. 4, 2014, pp. 306-308. *Wiley Library Online,* doi: 10.1111/birt.12134. Accessed 20 May 2016.

2.
Beyond the Birth Room

Building a Placenta-Positive Culture

AMY STENZEL

THE PLACENTA IS OUR FIRST RELATIONSHIP. It is the literal
site of connection between our new body and that of our
mother. In the watery world of the unborn, the placenta beats out
an ancient rhythm, tethering us to life itself. Yet from a Western
medical perspective, there is nothing sacred about the placenta at
all. It is merely a hunk of blood and tissue, destined for incineration
soon after a baby takes her first breaths. The primal connection
is abruptly cut off, with little regard to the physical and symbolic
repercussions to the individual child or to culture at large. In this
chapter, I attempt to uncover the importance of honouring the
placenta and to rediscover what is lost when these integral organs
are tossed aside. I argue that a shift toward alternate placental
rituals can begin to heal our overmedicalized society through the
valuation of maternity, womanhood, and caring relationships. It
is my firm belief that the placenta, as a literal and metaphorical
site of connection, must be reconceptualized in Western culture to
build healthier human communities from the start of life.

PLACENTAL SYMBOLISM AND FEMINIST DISCOURSE

The hospital environment is not a place for symbolic reasoning.
Bodies are being rushed in, stitched up, and reconfigured based
solely on functional needs, and, in most cases, that makes sense.
In an emergency, seconds matter, and no surgeon is going to use
those precious seconds to consider the symbolic and cultural implications behind his scalpel. The problem arises when we force the

experience of childbirth into this specialized system. Most births are not fast, and most are not an emergency. Birth, in essence, is the act of life bringing, not lifesaving. The symbolic understandings of childbirth have implications far beyond the hospital doors, going on to influence larger cultural imaginings of womanhood and personhood. Adrienne Rich argues that "what we bring to childbirth is nothing less than our entire socialization as women," (182) and the reverse is also true. What we learn from childbirth goes on to influence the future socialization of women and girls. From personal birth stories to advertisements for hospital birthing suites, the culture of birth is reproduced in greater society. However, as feminist Immogen Tyler points out, "within the cacophony [sic] of maternal publicity, only certain kinds of maternal experience can be communicated and heard" (5). The mainstream story of childbirth in the West is one of fear and panic, directly linked to the regulating logic of hospital care.

The few feminist scholars who have considered the alienation of medicalized birth have all identified the need for a new symbolic language around the process. Emily Martin in particular has written about this process. She argues that "metaphors, once chosen as the basis for description of physiological events, [have] profound impacts for the way in which ... the system will be perceived" (42). She concludes that "new key metaphors, core symbols of birth, [may] capture what we do not want to lose about birth" (157). The need for symbolic awareness is clear for birthing women, but the influence of birth symbology reaches all of us, whether we plan to birth children or not.

Birth is an unpopular topic among contemporary feminist theorists, which is due, in part, to the desire to deconstruct the image of women as domestic beings. Although women's issues outside of the home certainly deserve attention, I agree with Immogen Tyler that "birth [is] a vital site for contemporary feminist thought and practice" (6). This is particularly pertinent when considering the placenta. In a personal interview with Amanda Johnson, founder of the International Placenta and Postpartum Association, she argues that "when someone is denying a woman something that came from her body for their own agenda, or when a woman is meant to feel ashamed or gross for something natural, it definitely becomes a feminist issue." That the placenta is ignored in feminist discourse represents not a lack of importance but a certain ignorance to the larger inequities that play out in this specific bodily moment.

In "Amazing Placenta," placenta specialist Sarah Buckley says the following:

> placental symbolism is everywhere in our culture, from the handbags that we carry—holding our money, datebooks, and other items of survival—to the soft toys that we cram into our babies' cribs. Some believe that much of our culture's discontent and our urge to accumulate possessions—including all of the aforementioned—come from the traumatic loss of our first possession: our placenta. (55)

If Buckley is correct, the symbolic resonance of placenta ritual influences much more than the birth experience. The culture around the placenta may be perpetuating rampant Western consumerism, body exploitation, and the patriarchal control of all women. Some argue that most women do not care about the placenta, so theorists should not either. However, "very little research has been carried out to better understand women's views of the placenta [and] what meanings they attach to it" (Fannin 301). Of course, this is not the first time that medical science has ignored women's lived experience. Barbara Katz Rothman has written extensively about the way women are symbolically removed from the birthing process. She argues that "the alienation of the woman from birth, and more fundamentally from the body, is ... the most important and consistent theme in modern obstetrics" (105).

CUTTING THE CORD: MAINSTREAM PLACENTA NARRATIVES

Although Rothman does not focus on the placenta, she does highlight the role of medical culture in the establishment of the mother-baby connection. She criticizes Western modes of birth for ignoring that "a baby enters the world already in a relationship, a physical, social and emotional relationship with the woman in whose body it was nurtured" (57). Indeed, when reflecting on her own birth experiences, Adrienne Rich surmises that "the very nature of the mother-child bond may depend on the degree of contact in the first hours and days of the child's life" (180). Numerous studies have shown Rich's suspicion to be true. Many experts advocate for breastfeeding and skin-to-skin contact to support the mother-baby bond, so why is so little consideration being given to the placenta?

It would seem natural to value the placenta, given its vital and primary role in connecting mother and baby. However, when taking a closer look at the mainstream medical discussion of the placenta, it seems that this deep connection is itself what disturbs the status quo. Ethicist Eva-Maria Simms describes "the placenta [as a] phenomen[on] of female human embodiment that challenge[s] the philosophical notion of separate, sovereign subjects independent of other human beings" (263). Put simply, the placenta disrupts the Western values of masculine individuality and self-reliance, so important to our governing structure. Scientist Y.W. Loke states that "the placenta occupies a position midway between the baby and mother, in a kind of *'no-man's land'*" (6, emphasis mine). On a symbolic level, the placenta is a space outside of masculinity, where *no man* has power. The placental link of mother and child comes to represent the female power of life-giving, which threatens patriarchal narratives.

In response to the threat to power embodied in the placenta, Western medical discourse attempts to minimize and even demonize the organ. One example of this is the tradition of a male or father cutting the umbilical cord immediately upon birth. This is a symbolically resonant act, separating the baby from feminine dependency and bringing him into the masculinist culture of the public. Although this is likely not the conscious intention of the new father, the underlying symbolic act still functions to claim the infant as separate from the mother. Another example of the symbolic disempowerment of the placenta is found in the mainstream clinical language surrounding it. Many medical writings refer to the placenta in cold, mechanical terms. Loke, for example, writes that the baby uses "the placenta via the umbilical cord like a jump lead to plug into the mother's battery while its own is flat" (1). Even more degrading than the mechanistic descriptions of the placenta are the many depictions of the placenta as violent and pathological. Loke goes on to state that the placenta "defies conventional biological classification. Is it a transplant, a cancer, a parasite?" (223). Because he cannot make sense of the placenta within the masculinist medical construction of the body, Loke vilifies the life-giving organ as a deadly invader.

This mode of discourse is surprisingly common in the scientific community. In an interview with the *New York Times*, Dr. Susan Fisher says that "it looks like some monster thing from the deep chasms of the sea," when describing the placenta (qtd. in Grady). This dramatic disempowerment of the placenta can even be traced back through history. The artists and scientists of the Renaissance were seemingly biased against placental representation. Although "famed for his critical eye for detail in all his anatomical illustrations, Leonardo curiously left out the placenta" in his famous drawing of a child in the womb (Loke 3). These tropes are routinely seen in action. Obstetric textbooks show either a cold, minimal description of the placenta or, alternately, a monstrous analysis of its invasive and unknowable nature.

CHANGING THE SYMBOLS, CHANGING THE STORY

These are the messages that we are sending women about their bodies. The vilification or complete erasure of the placenta in birthing practice is co-constructive of the wider acceptance of violence practised on female bodies. However, there are alternatives. Some women are choosing to reject the standard placenta protocol to create their own rituals that celebrate the mother-baby connection. Anthropologist Melissa Cheyney argues that the "celebration of the placenta communicate[s] important messages to mothers about the sufficiency of their bodies and the sacredness of their birth experiences" (539). Her findings are consistent with the experiences reported by mothers and midwives who have participated in alternate placenta rituals. Placenta educator Sister Morningstar states that "I felt a glow in my heart to return to women, and some young men, a simple path of honoring placenta wisdom" (27). Revitalizing respect for the placenta simply feels right for many people.

Many non-Western cultures have always held positive placental rituals, and they can provide a model for a reimagined placental culture within the Western system. Sarah Buckley explores the nuances of these global practices, which range from simple ceremonial burial to more complex uses for the placenta and its parts. In Turkey, for example, the placenta is traditionally buried, but the final location of the umbilical cord is thought to determine the traits of the child. The cord "may be buried in the courtyard of a mosque, if the parents wish the child to be devout later in life;" if they want to child to be "well educated, they may throw the cord over a schoolyard wall" (Buckley, "Placenta Rituals" 58). The placenta has been used as medicine in traditional Chinese culture and even likely played a role in the political power of pharaohs of Ancient Egypt. There is a long history of placental ritual, which celebrates the power of the birthing body across cultures.

Both old and new placenta rituals are helping women to rediscover power in their birthing experiences. Placenta art has a growing following in the West, and a handful of professionals can be hired to create personal placenta prints, dried umbilical cord keepsakes, and even more. Lotus Birth, the practice of allowing the placenta and newborn to separate without intervention, is also growing in popularity. In the introduction to Shivam Rachana's book *Lotus Birth*, Sarah Buckley describes the practice as "an exquisite ritual that has enhanced the magic of the early post-natal days." She sees a positive impact of lotus birth on her own family, saying: "I notice an integrity and self-possession with my lotus-born children, and I believe that lovingness, cohesion, attunement to Mother Nature, and trust and respect for the natural order have all been imprinted on our family by our honouring of the placenta."

MAKING THE SHIFT, ONE BIRTH AT A TIME

Whether lotus birthing, placenta printing, or some other placental ritual is practised, the overall result is a restored sense of honour for women's bodies and the ongoing connection between mother and child. These rituals stand in direct contrast to the masculinist medical rhetoric that currently dominates the placenta conversation. Emily Martin describes medical culture as "a powerful system of socialization which exacts conformity as the price of participation" (13). Defying this conformity demanded by medicalized birth structures has the potential to break down problematic views of women's bodies.

Deciding on an alternate placenta practice may seem like a small, personal choice, but the impact of these choices should not be underestimated. By claiming her placenta as a symbol of power, a mother is rejecting the structures that oppress all female bodies. Her personal choice is also a political statement, demanding respect for her connection with her baby and for her ability to choose what is best for both of them. As Adrienne Rich writes, the "process of childbirth [is] a continuum, interwoven inextricably with the entire spectrum of a woman's life" (180). A culture that honours the placenta could provide strength for women, mothers, and non-mothers, throughout their lives.

WORKS CITED

Buckley, Sarah J. "The Amazing Placenta." *Mothering*, vol. 131, 2005, pp. 50-55.

Buckley, Sarah. Introduction. *Lotus Birth*, by Shivam Rachana, Greenword Press, 2000, http://archive.is/n7Lqj. Accessed 13 Apr. 2016.

Buckley, Sarah J. "Placenta Rituals and Folklore from Around the World." *Midwifery Today With International Midwife*, vol. 80, 2006, pp. 58-59.

Cheyney, M. "Reinscribing the Birthing Body: Homebirth as Ritual Performance." *Medical Anthropology Quarterly*, vol. 25, no.4, 2011, pp. 519-542.

Fannin, Maria. "Placental Relations." *Feminist Theory*, vol. 15, no. 3, 2014, pp. 289-306.

Grady, Denise. "The Push to Understand the Placenta." *New York Times*, 14 July 2014, https://www.nytimes.com/2014/07/15/health/the-push-to-understand-the-placenta.html?_r=0. Accessed 20 Apr 2016.

Johnson, Amanda. Personal interview. 5 May 2015.

Loke, Y.W. *Life's Vital Link: The Astonishing Role of the Placenta*. Oxford University Press, 2013.

Martin, Emily. *The Woman in the Body: A Cultural Analysis of Reproduction*. Beacon Press, 1987.

MorningStar, Sister. "Honoring Placenta Wisdom." *Midwifery Today*, vol. 109, 2014, pp. 26-27.

Rothman, Barbara Katz. *Recreating Motherhood*. Rutgers University Press, 2000.

Simms, Eva-Maria. "Eating One's Mother: Female Embodiment in a Toxic World." *Environmental Ethics*, vol. 31, no. 3, 2009, pp. 263-277.

Tyler, Imogen. "Introduction: Birth." *Feminist Review*, vol. 93, 2009, pp. 1-6.

3.
Slightly Inappropriate, but Really Brilliant

NICOLE LINK-TROEN

M Y MOTHER HAD SEVEN C-SECTIONS. Caesarean surgery has defined all of my life, starting with my own likely unnecessary Caesarean that then necessitated all the ones done upon my mother's body thereafter. My birth was her first, and her last occurred when I was sixteen. She told me that we were rather brutally separated for the first ten hours of my life because my body temperature just wouldn't regulate, or so they said. She was a college drop-out, a very young and unwed mother in the Deep South. Breastfeeding, also rather predictably, did not go well.

This separation from her first baby made my mother stronger for her other babies. It made her speak up and insist that she stay with her babies at a time when mothers and babies were still routinely and regularly separated during the immediate postpartum and definitely after a Caesarean. The only sleep I allowed myself in the hospital after the birth of my first son was when my mother was there in the room, sitting on the couch, guarding the door like a Doberman. I knew she would not let anyone whisk my baby to the nursery while I slept.

By her fifth birth, my mother was so good at advocating for herself that an hour after surgery, she was in the NICU with her newborn. He was full term at ten pounds and three ounces and had to go for respiratory and cardiac difficulties, but no hospital protocols were going to keep them apart. I was twelve at the time and remember scrubbing in to go see my newest brother, my "baby" as it were. Those were the high points, the arrival of my siblings, with all the waiting finally over. What those doctors did not see and did not know was the day-to-day grind of domesticity. With each Caesarean, my mother was ordered more bedrest. There were more children to take care of, and with a father working, those tasks fell to me. She spent a cumulative total of three years on bedrest.

Women in hospital gowns, IV tubes, beeping machines, and the smell of sanitizers all create simultaneous feelings of both terror and comfort within me. I could, and did, blame my mother for continuing to have babies in such a difficult and dangerous way, and she does hold some responsibility for her choices. But now that I know more, I do think that the overarching continuous pathologization of birth by the obstetric community in the late 1980s and early 1990s is also to blame for my (and her) lived experience.

Only very recently in North America have midwives been able to get back into the birthing room, with a modicum of trust in women's bodies being restored to obstetrics. My own story as a birthing woman in the early twenty-first century is a reflection of the growing idea that birth is something that the human female body can do well and that the more the process is interfered with, the more likely further interventions will be needed.

Growing up around someone who was almost continually pregnant, on bedrest, or recovering from surgery all but ensured that I would find myself drawn to birth work. When I ventured into motherhood very shortly after college, I did not know what working in birth looked like. My midwives were my first introduction to the world of birth work, which supports and allows women to become empowered.

* * *

At only two-weeks pregnant, I called the first homebirth midwife I could find. We started with the first question I had.

"Can I keep my placenta, or do you have to remove it? I really want to bury it."

"Of course you can keep it! It's your placenta. Do whatever you want with it. I know women who cook it up and eat it."

"Well, I don't want to eat it. Just bury it."

"That's totally fine. Just be sure that you dig a deep enough hole that the roots have several inches of dirt between them and the placenta, otherwise the decay will be too harsh on the plant."

Seven months later, sitting in her office for a prenatal, I was uncontrollably weeping, yet again. We revisited the whole "to eat placenta or not to eat placenta" question and decided that perhaps I should take some preventative measures against developing a postpartum mood disorder. She adamantly suggested that I try placenta encapsulation.

When my own grandmother found out that I was planning to eat my placenta, her words were "You can't do that, honey. That's a sin! It's cannibalism, and I won't be able to speak to you!"

I did not blame her for her visceral rejection of the idea, since eating your placenta after giving birth is slightly inappropriate, but when considering the potential benefits, it is really brilliant, so I went for it. My grandmother has since come around after witnessing my postpartum recovery.

I had seen a placenta before at the age of ten, but only on a video of my cousin's accidentally unassisted homebirth. Until seeing that home video, I had assumed that the doctor cut the babies umbilical cord, and then just sort of pushed it back up inside the mother and then sewed her shut. (My mother talked a lot about this "sewing" part of birth.) Watching the video with my aunt, she said, "and here comes the placenta, that part was worse than birthing the baby."

Startled, I said, "The what?"

"The placenta," my aunt replied. "It's the alien jelly fish thing that grows with the baby. We're planning to bury it and plant a tree over it. It's in the freezer now."

This was my introduction to the magical placenta. I would not see another one until I saw my own, twelve years later.

The day of my son's birth, we transferred from home to the hospital because of moderate meconium and maternal fatigue after two days of labour. After a bag of IV fluid, I gave birth vaginally and unmedicated in the hospital, flanked by my husband, my midwife, and attended by her backing OB. Although I was terrified on the drive there, the smell of the hospital was astonishingly comforting to me, as it was imprinted in my brain as the place where babies are born safely. After the birth of the placenta, I remember asking my midwife for a piece of it, and the medical staff cringed a bit as she put a piece in my mouth anyway. When the placenta is warm, it is really not so bad raw. On the day that a person exits your body, eating a piece of placenta is one of the lesser weird things that you can do. I had hired an encapsulator to turn the bulk of the placenta into easy-to-take pills, and she came right away to encapsulate it in my kitchen.

Three months out from birth, I found myself unemployed, with no community, no car, no career, and a colicky baby. No amount of placenta pills can overcome all of that, but I do think that they helped us survive. I had a steady milk supply, had stopped bleeding extraordinarily fast, and had felt pretty stable those first weeks wintering with my newborn.

I knew those placenta pills held some magic, and I wanted to share that and make some freaking mom friends. I figured the best way to make mom friends was to be there when they became moms. At the time, I was a new mother with a three-month-old baby. But without a single friend to call and talk with about what I was going through—both the mental and physical changes that were happening to me—meant that I did suffer from a massive bout of postpartum anxiety. The problem: I had a bachelor's in history, a new baby, and no way to afford childcare to get a "real" job. All I had was this burning desire to meet other mothers and to be there for them—the way that I wished they would be there for me. In becoming a mother myself, I had learned so much about breastfeeding and birthing a baby, and I wanted to know more. I wanted to share that information with other women, and I wanted to support my family doing it.

When I broached the subject of becoming a placenta encapsulation specialist, I was met with a great deal of scepticism from my family, but I went for it anyway. I signed up for a placenta benefits course and started reading the relevant academic papers that covered placentophagy, and my mind sang![1] For the first time in months, I was on familiar ground, reading study after study and writing essays again. I still had a colicky baby, and breastfeeding was still a challenge, but the placenta encapsulation training gave me hope and purpose.

I sped through the coursework and felt like myself for the first time in over a year. Research articles, essays, and tests were all so wonderfully familiar that I knew that I was doing the right thing. In

March of 2010, within a week of completing training and putting my equipment together, the phone rang unexpectedly. It was my midwife. She said, "I have a placenta for you."

"Oh, really? Great! When is she due?"

"Too late for that! The baby's here. She was born last night. Mom had to transfer to the hospital and the placenta is still at home."

"Oh, woah, ok! I can come now."

And thus it began. An hour later, I was washing dishes in the new mom's kitchen, while her parents talked with me about growing avocados, of all things. The mother herself was miles away, trying to recover from a hemorrhage and perineal repair. Once all the dishes were done and the counters were cleaned and covered, I opened the Tupperware container and a slight wave of nausea went over me. That feeling quickly passed as I registered the familiar coppery smell of blood. I had seen and touched my own son's placenta a few months before, but this was different.

This was something I had never been privileged or privy to before, yet I was trusted to handle it. That part still gets me, that I am trusted. Every placenta must be processed perfectly, no mistakes, no exceptions. As the encapsulator, I have one shot. During my first encapsulation, I was nervous as anything, but I trusted my training, and it did not let me or my client down. As I drove away from that first house, I knew I was doing exactly what I was supposed to be doing for the first time in a long time.

During follow-up calls and emails, my clients often say something along the lines of "Thank you! You are awesome! I feel so good, these pills you made are amazing!"

"Nonsense." I reply. "You made the placenta, and, therefore, you made the pills. All I did was clean it up a bit. Every bite you took in your pregnancy, every cell you grew—YOU—your body made something perfect for you to use. And you made the decision to use it. Thank you for entrusting me with your placenta."

I knew that I would meet and make new friends through placenta encapsulation work and that did happen in fits and starts over the first several years. I worked hard to make connections with other mothers, and we traded childcare so I could encapsulate. I became pregnant with my second child in the second year of being an encapsulator. After the homebirth of my second son, my community had grown to such an extent that I was fully supported. People brought meals, kept me company, played with my older child, and we had so much fun. I took my placenta pills for that postpartum too, and I had a strong social support system and a stable career identity. My second birth and postpartum was all that I could have hoped for emotionally and physically.

What I did not know or expect when I started encapsulation services was that I had started a business. And that in addition to supporting new mothers, I would also be helping to support my family. I had no idea when I started that the public "placenta lady" identity would become who I am in my community or that it would give me so much joy. I do not typically take vacations, and if I do, it is never more than a few hours away so that we can return quickly if "the call" comes. It is a small sacrifice to pay to do the thing that I love. Working with placentas is both very limiting and also liberating; it is soul-fulfilling in a way that only new life and the immediate postpartum can be.

Working for new mothers is a privilege, and to continue to do it well I must be compensated fairly. When people first meet me and learn what I do, they assume that I am a fully attachment parenting, uber-crunchy, mega-hippie. They soon learn that I support mothers' choices whatever they may be and that I'm actually pretty mainstream. In reality, we are all doing our best and doing what works to get these children and ourselves through life. My clients come from all walks of life. I love listening to their stories and being there as they make their final transitions into parenthood.

Approximately 90 percent of my clients birth in the hospital. Since I start fresh, within forty-eight hours of birth, I very rarely get to meet the women that I work for. I have started doing postpartum doula work so that I can really get to know them and be there for them when they transition to being a new parent at home. Mostly, I find myself in all kinds of kitchens rinsing off a placenta with a newly minted grandmother standing next to me asking questions and a grandfather or two standing in the background making the exact same joke about how they are going to eat the placenta.

The grandmothers are honestly my favourite. They stand next to me, eager to help out, curious, and slightly grossed out. I start explaining about the placenta—the anatomy and functions—and

I also point out the tree of life imagery. Then, suddenly, it dawns on them, "This is my grandbaby's placenta. This is really cool. I grew a placenta too! Life is AMAZING! I did something amazing! My daughter/daughter-in-love did something AWESOME!"

So many women of older generations were not given the opportunity to see what they had created and were taught to disdain their placentas. It is my supreme joy to demystify the placenta for these wise women. Within a few days time, those grandmothers and their daughters then stand witness to the benefits and the power of the placenta capsules, and they tell their friends.

I do not expect validation for placentophagy from the medical community, and I certainly share their concerns over potential unknown risks. At this point in time, literally hundreds of mothers have tried placenta encapsulation and found positive results from it. Discounting those experiences with constant negativity and reaching for potential problems without supporting evidence is disheartening and smacks of the chronic disbelief concerning women's experiences that has so plagued women's health care. To be truly culturally sensitive to mothers who plan to consume their placentas, care providers must be familiar with the practice and not condemn it. Nor should they condone unsafe practices, such as improper preparation. The key is to ask questions, listen to women, and respect their choices. That is the heart and soul of working with new mothers successfully.

ENDNOTE

[1] I took the original placenta encapsulation coursework created by Jodi Selander of http://placentabenefits.info/ in February of 2010. The most up-to-date placenta benefits course is currently at http://placentacourse.com/.

4.
"I'm Just Going to Give You the Injection for the Placenta"

Active Management of the Third Stage and the Myth of Informed Consent

ALYS EINION

STANDARD PRACTICE IN THE WESTERN and biomedical con-text is to encourage the use of oxytocic drugs to facilitate and speed up the "third stage of labour" (the delivery of the placenta), typically through an injection. This critical chapter examines the history of this practice, its impact on women's birth experiences, and the language that is used to direct women toward this practice rather than toward a natural or physiologic placental delivery.[1]

I examine the culture of midwifery from the perspective of the United Kingdom and the nature of risk, which affects this culture. I examine and explore the concept of informed choice as well as the rhetoric of control, which alienates women from their own bodies and, therefore, their own placentas.

True choice in maternity care, though central to policy and prac-tice discourses for twenty-three years, remains the holy grail of childbearing mostly in principle. As most midwives would admit, exercising choice during pregnancy and birth is at best a challenge and at worst, a well-disguised myth. Regan et al. describe choice as "problematic" because

> it assumes that women's birthing choices are a matter of unrestricted preferences. However, that assumption denies the profound cultural and symbolic significance of birth and fails to account for how social discourse influences women's knowledge about birth and the subsequent choices they make. (172)

Since women rarely experience true informed choice, a midwife is placed in an invidious, not to say precarious, position. Midwives are required to act as advocates for women, in their role aligned with a woman-centred approach to care. In this, the maintenance of unequal power relationships results in midwives offering women limited choices, even as they supposedly act in their best interests.

PLACENTA DELIVERY AND THE FRAMING OF CHOICE

The placenta—that life-giving, nurturing vital organ, glorious despite its impermanence—is treated within Western culture, medicine, and discourse as a waste product. The "third stage of labour," the period between the birth of the baby and the delivery of the placenta and membranes, is a point on the childbearing journey that is automatically medically managed within the UK, unless the birthing mother has exercised considerable effort in opting for no intervention. Intervention comes in the form of the intramuscular injection of an oxytocic agent—either Syntocinon or Syntometrine—at the birth of the anterior shoulder, or as soon afterwards as possible. The aim of this standard practice is to reduce the risk of postpartum haemorrhage by ensuring that the placenta and membranes are expelled swiftly and that the uterus contracts effectively over the placental bed. The placental bed is a large site for rapid haemorrhage, but the normal process following birth involves a rush of oxytocin that causes the uterus to contract tightly, compressing the placental site and stemming the flow of blood to that area.

In the absence of intervention, the expulsion of the placenta can take up to an hour or more. When the placenta is still in situ, partial separation of the placenta from the uterine wall can occur, resulting in haemorrhage while the placenta is still in utero, preventing the full contraction of the uterus. Thus, what is known as "active management" of the third stage also involves the use of controlled cord traction by a midwife or doctor to expedite delivery of the placenta, after they observe for signs of separation, signified by lengthening of the cord and a small gush of fresh blood. In physiological management, skin-to-skin contact and early breastfeeding encourage the release of oxytocin, which enables this process to occur naturally. The birthing mother will typically feel a sensation of something in the vagina or an urge to push, and will birth the placenta herself as she did her baby.

It is interesting to reflect on my eighteen years as a midwife in the UK and to recall how easily, in such a blasé manner, I, like many of my colleagues, simply checked that the box had been ticked in the labour plan, confirming that consent had been given for the injection for the third stage of labour, and then smoothly stated "I'm just going to give you the injection." After completing my degree, I was a hospital midwife, so I was rarely involved in that decision-making process. In the UK, when working in a hospital setting, I only saw women during labour or after birth, or if they were admitted to the antenatal ward with complications. However, from time to time, a client would not have given prior consent, and I would have the chance to discuss the choice with them. True to the culture of the time, I framed this decision the way I had been taught to, the way I had observed other midwives doing so. The option was to have a shorter period of time between baby and placenta and reduce the risk of bleeding, or to wait and see, which could make it much longer before the woman could have her tea and toast, shower, and take the next step along the journey that is the transition to motherhood. Even as I did so, I knew that although I was ostensibly offering choice, I was framing that choice in such a way as to make the injection the most attractive option. It removed some of the stress of the situation and expedited the labour "conveyor belt." This was an enculturated phenomenon, which pushed midwives to efficiently move women through labour and birth and after birth, to swiftly accomplish all the necessary tasks required to transfer the woman and her infant to the postnatal ward, thus freeing up the birth room for the next client. That joyous time when the mother first meets her infant is subject to institutional timetables that hurry her through the bonding process. My memories of that time were of the pressure from colleagues and the ward manager to get her to the ward as quickly as possible.

Abhyankar et al. show that decision making is affected by the way in which information is presented to the receiver. This is evident in the way that risk information is presented, particularly relating to the explicit information to be used for evaluation. As a consequence, "different presentations of the same situation can therefore induce people to form markedly different mental representations, which, in turn, lead to different choices" (2). What is significant about considering the choice to have intervention for the delivery of the placenta is that midwives are taught to frame this choice in such a way as to minimize any negative aspects of what the system sees as the most desirable outcome: an actively managed third stage. This is apparently common in healthcare, as benefits are emphasized and risks are minimized in the process of positioning "an option as the only sensible choice" (Abhyankar et al. 2). And although I cannot claim to have witnessed a huge range of midwives addressing this aspect of their role, my experience, both personal and vicarious through the eyes of my students, suggests that this is very much the case within midwifery in the UK.

Why do hospitals and midwives see this as preferable? The first reason is the evidence, as reinforced by the World Health Organisation (WHO): it helps to reduce the risk of haemorrhage. The WHO recommends that such drugs be available for women worldwide. This is an important and inescapable fact, but one that should be considered in context. Yes, these drugs should be available. Yes, women should be offered them, and, where necessary, they should be used to address the issue of postpartum haemorrhage. Women in the UK have the privilege of being attended by skilled personnel, who are trained to respond to any signs of postpartum haemorrhage. These personnel, primarily midwives, have access to all the requisite drugs for treating a haemorrhage. Why then should women not have a true choice between what may be the only intervention in their labour and continuing with an entirely natural, self-determined birth experience?

Midwives are required to practise in a way that places the woman, the client, at the centre of all decision making. In reality, this "woman-centred" care is a term that is bandied about with little real meaning for many midwives, particularly as they continue to wield their specialist knowledge as a means of maintaining power over the woman, thereby powerfully influencing the decision-making process. However, midwives themselves are also oppressed by the technocratic and medical model of birth in which they practice and within which they are required to work, according to evidence-based guidelines. The limitations of that evidence are significant. Midwives can only work with the best available evidence, and when the gold standard of evidence is defined as the "randomized controlled trial,"[2] they find that the concept of woman-centred, individualised care has been erased from the clinical equation. There are studies that focus on the experience of women, on the holistic dimensions of that experience, and on the "soft" side of practice—the humanistic, artful, and highly personal nature of pregnancy and birth (Darra and Murphy; Crowther et al.). However, these have little effect on the way that policy is created or on the writing of protocols, which limits the autonomy and decision making ability of the midwife herself.

FIGURATIVE AUTONOMY

Midwives in the UK have, thus far, retained their autonomous status as practitioners in their own right, as experts in normal birth. But in this area of maternity care, as in so many others, that autonomy appears figurative. Working within the National Health Service, the midwife is required to follow guidelines, which are more like law than a suggested framework for optimizing practice. Although practice still focuses on the traditional active management process for delivering the placenta, there is growing evidence that challenges this routine approach. Two randomized controlled trials, for example, show that although the use of uterotonic drugs is associated with a lower rate of postpartum haemorrhage, controlled cord traction is not (Gulmezoglu et al.; Deneux-Tharawux et al.).

In order for midwives to retain their position in the medical hierarchy, they must adhere to both the requirements of the UK Nursing and Midwifery Council (NMC) and of their employer. They have a subordinate position in this hierarchy, in which they are, often unknowingly, as oppressed as their clients. Midwives are often limited in expressing the full scope of their role for the benefit of women. The majority of UK maternity services use the guidelines from the National Institute of Health and Care Excellence (NICE) as a means of evidencing their care provision and protecting themselves from litigation. Based on NICE guidelines, midwives recommend active management of the third stage, and present the injection as something routine and minimal in its effects. Yet the drug's effects are significant: women experience nausea and vomiting, and a disinclination toward holding and feeding their babies.

According to the online electronic Medicines Compendium (eMC)—which provides information on the mode of action, cautions, contraindications and undesirable effects of Syntometrine—nausea, vomiting and rash can occur, along with other effects. This source also states the following: "ergometrine derivatives are excreted in breast milk but in unknown amounts. There is no specific data available for elimination of ergometrine partitioned in breast-milk. Ergometrine can inhibit prolactin secretion and in turn can suppress lactation, so its repeated use should be avoided." The same source also lists a range of potential drug interactions and other adverse effects, few of which seem to be discussed with women as part of the decision-making process.

A study by Amy Brown and Sue Jordan finds an association between the use of prophylactic uterotonics and a reduction in the duration of breastfeeding. The authors recommend more random-ized trials of management of the third stage of labour, and also argue that those mothers who have been given a uterotonic should have more support with breastfeeding. It is interesting to note that in this study there is no differentiation between Syntometrine and Syntocinon, despite what is stated above about its effects. Other research shows that using synthetic oxytocin affects the physiology of the hormones of lactation (Leng et al), but some of this research also shows that exogenous oxytocin may enhance positive mood in some women (Jonas et al.). Brown and Jordan argue that synthetic oxytocin interrupts the natural hormone balance for breastfeed-ing, whereas Jonas et al. suggest that it compensates for the lack of natural oxytocin caused by epidural analgesia. Therefore, the evidence base appears mixed.

SUPPORTING PHYSIOLOGY

Conversely, the physiology of birth can be enhanced through the provision of a supportive environment and care practices that promote the normal functioning of the autonomic nervous system and the normal neuro-endocrine release mechanisms for oxytocin. Saxton et al. argue that "physiological oxytocin release is much more effective in maintaining eutony and eulochia compared with the injection of artificial oxytocin" because of the inherent pulsatile release of a woman's own oxytocin, which works more effectively than artificially administered oxytocin ("Effects" 253). They discuss the complex interactions between the environment of birth, the woman's feelings and psychological environment, and the need for a trusting relationship with a midwife. The authors conclude that "all women and babies should be enabled and supported to have immediate and prolonged skin-to-skin contact and breastfeeding at birth ... so that ... the risk of posttpartum haemorrhage is minimised" (253).

The findings of a Cochrane review show that there is insufficient evidence that breastfeeding or nipple stimulation reduces the incidence of postpartum haemorrhage, but this is an issue of lack of evidence rather than any indication that it would not be effective (Abedi et al.). A study in New Zealand by Davis et al. shows that in low-risk women, "women receiving active management of the third stage of labor experienced a twofold increase in the risk of blood loss greater than 1,000 mL compared with those having a physiological third stage of labor" (104). A cohort study by Saxton et al. also shows that breastfeeding immediately after birth and skin-to-skin contact between mother and infant may reduce rates of postpartum haemorrhage ("Does Skin-to-Skin").

However, the overwhelming weight of evidence is in favour of active management as a means of reducing postpartum haemorrhage and length of the second stage of labour (WHO). But the question remains: why give a drug routinely when it could be employed after birth in the light of any signs of haemorrhage? The indications for the use of Syntometrine, for example on the eMC, are "the active management of the third stage of labour (as a means to promote separation of the placenta and to reduce blood loss), or routinely, following the birth of the placenta, to prevent or treat postpartum haemorrhage."

One of the reasons that midwives may not fully inform women of the facts before supporting informed decision making could be lack of confidence in not only providing the right information but in supporting women to birth their placentas naturally. Expectant management of the third stage is generally seen as the alternative to what is viewed as the mainstream approach. This is only recommended when there is no use of induction or augmentation of labour, and no epidural anaesthesia or any other indications of higher risk for postpartum haemorrhage (Begley et al., "Irish and New Zealand"). The benefits of expectant management have been highlighted by a Cochrane review of evidence. This review provides a balanced exploration of risks and benefits, and argues that women should be able to make a well-informed choice about this part of their care (Begley et al., "Active versus Expectant"). Interestingly and importantly, this review shows that the randomized trials that compare active versus expectant management took place in clinical areas in which midwives were not accustomed to supporting women with a physiological third stage. The women involved in the trials often had exogenous oxytocin during labour, which would then affect the physiology of the third stage. Expertise and confidence may be an issue.

Another reason for midwives not offering choice is that the culture of midwifery, particularly in the UK, does not truly support women who make well-informed choices because these choices may disrupt the status quo. The birth environment for the majority of births is a medically and artificially constructed environment, one in which midwives are socialized into supporting and maintaining through their initial education (Einion). Midwives occupy a position of authority in this environment and strive to maintain that position, despite the erosion of their role and autonomy within a litigious society (Hood et al.). But the precariousness of their position brings about a widespread submission to and compliance with a medically dominated culture, which, in turn, influences the births of the majority of women in the UK and in similar Westernized cultures.

I observe and hear discussed practices that I find inimical to the very nature of midwifery identity, which includes a culture of leaving labour-room doors routinely open and criticizing idealistic student midwives for wanting to shut the door. Offering privacy, safety, and security for women is fully aligned with every aspect of the role of the midwife. Offering informed choice within a supportive, egalitarian relationship and a positive-care environment is also central to midwives' work. However, a midwife cannot do this if she does not work in an environment that supports her to offer true informed choice. I write from a privileged position: I am paid to read extensively, explore the evidence, and critique the dominant discourses and practices of my profession. Midwives working within an oppressive culture and system do not always have such a luxury, and are so pressured by workload and time constraints that it leaves them little liberty or energy to do the reading and take up the cause that will result in any change to that system. We are, very effectively, kept powerless.

BEING WITH WOMEN

I became a midwife in order to be with women and to address critical, crucial, and challenging questions. I became a midwife to advocate for women's rights, equality, and autonomy during pregnancy and childbearing. During that process of becoming and throughout my career, my utter and complete confidence in the ability of women to bear children naturally has never wavered, and has only been confirmed over time by a deeper understanding of the science and the biological marvel that is the human body. As Saxton et al. show, the role of the midwife lies in "optimising the woman's reproductive physiology," as it is the midwife who supports the woman, manages the birth environment, and supports the way she copes with labour, birth, and the arrival of her baby ("Effects" 253). That midwives often struggle to achieve this, or become so inured to medical management of labour that they forget these fundamentals, is the strongest indictment of the maternity care system.

It is clear from even the small amount of literature explored during this discussion that there is a dissonance between the provision of woman-centred midwifery care with true partnership and collaborative decision making, and the processes and procedural norms by which maternity care is defined and delivered. The placenta is a wondrous organ, and the entire birth is an event in which women can locate and maintain autonomy, confidence, and a new and deeper understanding of their reproducing selves. Midwives who respect the placenta and its passage from the uterus—signifying the completion of its role and signifying the moment of change when baby becomes self as distinct from maternal body—promote and support the sense of awe and wonder that should surround the whole birth experience. We continue to successfully advocate for women having the birth they want. It is time also to advocate for their choice, autonomy, and decision making in relation to their placentas in equal measure.

There is no doubt that we should be actively preventing risk wherever possible when caring for women and babies. But taking this debate down to its most fundamental level, we should also not routinely administer an intervention without offering true choice. It is the role of the midwife, therefore, to become fully informed and share that information with their clients without prejudice. This includes the information about the negative, potentially harmful effects of routinized practice. If more women understood the rationale behind some delivery room practices, and truly understood that all decision making is a process of weighing risks and benefits within the limitations of scientific and experiential knowledge, they may be better able to engage with their midwives and develop that trusting relationship that is the core of a positive birth experience.

ENDNOTES

[1]There is an ever-widening birth discourse and rhetoric that utilizes a range of terms— including physiological and physiologic, normal, and natural—which are designed to indicate a normative, biologically unhindered process without medical intervention.

[2]The randomized controlled trial is a largescale scientific study carried out within strict parameters, in which interventions are tested by having a randomized sample of individuals be allocated to receive an intervention or not. This allows for a scientific evaluation of the effects of interventions versus no intervention. It is considered the most scientifically rigorous means of researching the effectiveness of modern healthcare practices but cannot be used to measure all aspects of healthcare.

WORKS CITED

Abedi, Parvin, et al. "Breastfeeding or Nipple Stimulation for Reducing Postpartum Haemorrhage in the Third Stage of Labour." *Cochrane Database of Systematic Reviews,* Issue 1, 2016, Art. No. D=CD010845. *NCBI,* doi: 10.1002/14651858.CD10845.pub.2.

Abhyanar, Purva, et al. "Framing Options as Choice or Opportunity: Does the Frame Influence Decisions?" *Medical Decision Making,* vol. 34, no. 5, 2014, pp. 567-582.

Begley, Cecily M. et al. "Irish and New Zealand Midwives' Expertise in Expectant Management of the Third Stage of Labour: the 'MEET' study." *Midwifery,* vol. 28, 2012, pp. 733-739.

Begley, Cecily M. et al. "Active Versus Expectant Management for Women in the Third Stage of Labour." *Cochrane Database of Systematic Reviews,* 2010, Art. No. CD007412. *Wiley,* doi: 10.1002/14651858.DC007412.pub2.

Brown, Amy, and Sue Jordan. "Active Management of the Third Stage of Labor May Reduce Breastfeeding Duration Due to Pain and Physical Complications." *Breastfeeding Medicine,* vol. 9, no. 10, 2014, pp. 494-502.

Crowther, Susan, et al.. "The Joy at Birth: An Interpretive Hermeneutic Literature Review." *Midwifery,* vol. 30, no. 4, 2014, pp. e157-e165.

Darra, Susanne, and Fiona Murphy. "Coping and Help in Birth: An Investigation into 'Normal' Childbirth as Described by New Mothers and their Attending Midwives." *Midwifery,* vol. 40, 2016, pp. 18-25.

Deneux-Tharaux, Catherine, et al. "Effect of Routine Controlled Cord Traction as Part of the Active Management of the Third Stage of Labour on Postpartum Haemorrhage: Multicentre Randomised Controlled Trial (TRACOR)." *British Medical Journal,* vol. 246, 2013, pp. f1541.

Einion, Alys. "What Have they Become?: Narrative Analysis of Student Learning Journals." International Conference on Normal Birth, June 2015, Lake District, UK. Conference Paper.

Electronic Medical Compendium (eMC). "Syntometrine® 500 micrograms/5 IU Solution for Injection." *Electronic Medical Compendium, United Kingdom.* 16 Jan. 2016, https://www.

medicines.org.uk/emc/medicine/135. Accessed April 2016.

Gulmezoglu, A. Metin et al. "Active Management of the Third Stage of Labour with and Without Controlled Cord Traction: A Randomised, Controlled, Non-inferiority Trial." *Lancet*, vol. 379, 2012, pp. 1721-1727.

Hood, Laraine, et al. "A Story of Scrutiny and Fear: Australian Midwives' Experiences of an External Review of Obstetric Services, Being Involved with Litigation and the Impact on Clinical Practice." *Midwifery*, vol. 26, no. 3, 2010, pp. 268-285.

Jonas, Wibke, et al. "Influence of Oxytocin or Epidural Analgesia on Personality Profile in Breastfeeding Women: A Comparative Study." *Archives of Women's Mental Health,* vol. 11, no. 5-6, 2008, pp. 335-345.

Leng, Gareth, Simone L. Meddle, and Alison J. Douglas. "Oxytocin and the Maternal Brain." *Current Opinion in Pharmacology,* vol. 8, no. 6, 2008, pp. 731-734.

Nursing and Midwifery Council. *The Code: Professional Standards of Practice and Behaviour for Nurses and Midwives.* NMC, 2015.

Regan, Mary, et al. "Choice? Factors that Influence Women's Decision Making for Childbirth." *The Journal of Perinatal Education,* vol. 22, no. 3, 2013, pp. 171-180.

Saxton, Anne, et al. "Effects of Skin-to-Skin Contact and Breastfeeding at Birth on the Incidence of PPH: A Physiologically Based Theory." *Women and Birth,* vol. 27, no.4, 2014, pp. 250-253.

Saxton, Anne, et al. "Does Skin-to-Skin Contact and Breastfeeding at Birth Affect the Rate of Primary Postpartum Haemorrhage: Results of a Cohort Study." *Midwifery,* vol. 31, no. 11, 2015, pp. 1110-1117.

World Health Organisation. "WHO Recommendations for Active Management of the Third Stage of Labour," WHO, 2014, http://apps.who.int/iris/bitstream/10665/119831/1/WHO_RHR_14.18_eng.pdf. Accessed 25 May 2016.

5.
"Placental Waste"

Wild Boys, Blood-Clot Boys,
and Long-Teeth Boys

BARBARA ALICE MANN

WORLDWIDE, WESTERN MEDICINE'S cavalier attitude toward and treatment of placentae and umbilici as "waste material" causes great distress to Indigenous peoples (Njikam 15). This includes the matriarchal cultures of Turtle Island (Indigenous North and Central America), whose women are still trying to get Western medical personnel to realize that disrespectfully handled placentae can lead to "Wild Boys," "Blood-Clot Boys," and "Long-Teeth Boys," who are unbalanced enough to wreak considerable harm on the environment and the people.

Apparently, though, we are just superstitious Indians. Our traditional reverence for, and postnatal care of, the placentae and umbilici were even outlawed by the U.S. federal government as part of its all-out war on Indigenous culture, looking to force Indigenous assimilation to Euro-Christian cultural norms. Full rights to practise Indigenous traditions were restored only in 1978, with certain states continuing the fight until the U.S. Supreme Court removed that option from them, which forced Congress fully to guarantee Indigenous rights in 1993 (Mann, *Spirits of Blood* 17-21; "Native Americans" 139-148; "Ending the Ban" 291-304).[1]

These restorations were too late for me when I gave birth to my beautiful daughter in 1972. Then, it was still against federal law to practice or explicate Indigenous cultural ways. However, when my daughter birthed her own exquisite daughter in 2002, she was able to save her daughter's umbilical stump for proper care, even though the afterbirth was thoughtlessly tossed by the medical staff while we, the family, were still making sure that she was all right, given her type 1 diabetes and her disastrous multiple sclerosis. I was about to bead the traditional cord pouch, when a Shawnee clan mother anticipated me, gifting my daughter with a sumptuously beaded turtle pouch, in which she placed my grand-daughter's stump.

To understand the complex, Indigenous treatment and tradition surrounding placentae and umbilici, the reader must first realize that everything on Turtle Island falls into one or the other half of the Twinned Cosmos. The Blood half, also referenced as the water half, relates to things of Mother Earth. The Breath half, sometimes called the air half, pertains to things of Brother Sky. The two are properly complements: there is no Manichean dichotomy of warring polarities going on here, outside of missionary mangling of our traditions! Instead, balancing the halves is the life-long obligation of all material in the cosmos, for everything has consciousness and balancing duties of some kind (Mann, *Spirits of Blood*). The mothers and brothers of sky and earth reflect the primary male-female relationship in Indigenous America—the Brother-Sister bond—in which the elder male of the family is the mother's brother, not her child's biological father. Some nations, mostly Plains peoples, refer to the sky half of the cosmos as "Grandfather," but he is *not* a god, and he is *not* a husband. He is a maternal great uncle.

Immersed in their own patriarchal, one-size-fits-all traditions, however, Euro-scholars, out "collecting" Indigenous traditions, simply did not grasp the Twinship distinctions that their Indigenous "informants" were drawing between Blood things and Breath things. Instead, anthropologists and ethnologists were so racially arrogant as not to concede unmuddled intelligence to their Indigenous interlocutors. Consequently, should something, *any*thing, not make sense to Westerners, scholars either discarded it as anomalous or, even more damagingly, they reinterpreted it in patriarchal terms that in no way reflected Indigenous matriarchal thinking on the matter—and we could not begin correcting them until 1978!

Notwithstanding, all Indigenous Americans honour their mother, the earth, in a multitude of ways, but some of the most powerful of those ways connect with childbirth, whose Blood-half placentae and umbilici require special attention, lest they go unbalanced, seeding havoc. The primary womb belongs, of course, to Mother Earth, Herself, so that the still potent placenta must be returned to Her by some means, for She alone can quell its excess energy. Burial in the ground always works. Caves, especially, are seen as the wombs of Mother Earth, with the Wyandots' Olentangy Caverns in Ohio traditionally viewed as fallopian tubes leading to the womb, as accessed by a fifty-five foot "vaginal" drop into the caverns (Mann, *Spirits of Blood* 165). Archaeologists are now thinking that one of the complex's chambers was a burial site.[2] Indeed, the whole Olentangy River basin was used, for at least two thousand years, as a series of cemetery sites (Dancey and Seeman 140-144). It is hardly surprising, then, that Ohio oral tradition holds that infants dying at birth were placed along with their afterbirth in pockets along the cavern's fallopian passages, as the mothers were reseating the child for rebirth. Indigenous America has its own philosophy of reincarnation, not at all connected with Eastern philosophies (Mann, *Spirits of Blood* 188-241). Live girls' afterbirth, particularly, would also be planted (buried) in this cave-womb, to be reabsorbed.

This said, the exact mode of afterbirth treatment varies depending on the nation and its landscape—Turtle Island is a vast continental complex with multiple climes and landforms—but all methods are variations on the idea that the placenta, with its associated umbilicus, hosts elemental Blood prowess, which must be quelled, lest it act on its own, outside of the womb, unmediated by its other half. These considerations determine how both the placentae and the umbilici are treated postnatally.

As with the living child, the sex of the placenta matters. Were a female placenta (Blood) to go to air (Breath) or a male placenta (Breath) go to water (Blood), results could be dire. Here, the anthropological record must be read gingerly, because among the points that Western scholars did not grasp was that among Indigenous Americans, men did male things and women did female things. Thus, men told men's stories. So when the anthropologists, nearly all male, went "collecting," they heard what applied to men only, but then extended it generally to include women as well.

As a result, anthropologists recorded Twinned methods of placental safekeeping as *alternatives*, not as Blood or Breath linked.

In recording that the placenta was put "in river," for instance, they did not realize that this was a proper placental burial for females only. And in claiming that the placenta was "thrown away any place," they missed that this indicated a male air-exposure burial, and one in a particular place, by the way (Stewart 332). Alternatively, scholars would observe just one method but assume that it pertained both to newborn boys and girls. Here, for example, they claimed that the Hupa people of California "split" open a young Douglas spruce tree to place both the placenta and the umbilical cord in the rift. Then they tied the tree back together, after which the child's progress and luck was determined by watching the fortunes of the growing spruce (Long 239).[3] Because trees, as lungs (of Mother Earth), fall into the air/Breath half of the cosmos, this custom was appropriate to male children's afterbirth, but it was given as if it applied to female placentae, too.

Instead, male placentae used Breath, whereas female placentae used Blood, methods of burial. In the extreme northwest of the continent, the Alaskan Ahtna people, who live along the Copper River, were said to have burned the placenta, a Breath-style burial, suggesting that this applied to male afterbirth, although some cultures, such as the patriarchal Mound Builders who date back as far as four thousand years ago, cremated for male and female (Long 236; Mann, *Native Americans*, 155-156, 167, 194-195; Mann and Fields, "A Sign in the Sky" 122-129). On the other end of sending off the placenta is the Blood (earth) water burial, which is safe for females but not for males. Consequently, putting the female placenta near fresh water is fairly commonplace, with some peoples even first wrapping it in a water-absorbent material to keep it moist (Curtis, *Portraits* 243). Zuñi maternal grandmothers, for example, carried the (female) afterbirth to the river, where they "buried" it (Stevenson 298).

Among the Kwakiutl of British Columbia, if the infant were female, then the placenta was Blood-buried at the high-water level of the tide (water is the amniotic fluid of Mother Earth), whereas if the infant were male, it was exposed to the open air (the Breath of Brother Sky) for ravens (Breath) to eat clean away. These burials also ensured that the girl child would grow up to be a good clam digger, whereas the boy child would grow up to enjoy the sharp, binocular hunting vision of the raven (Long 237). Importantly, both forms of Kwakiutl burials were safe because the placentae went to the cosmic half to which it belonged: women with water (Blood) and men with air (Breath).

In northern México (México being the Tail of Turtle Island), the Taramuhare people placed a hefty stone atop the buried placenta (Hrdlička 57, 61).[4] Stone over earth is very heavy Blood, replicating a cave burial. Failing a cave, women turned to other methods of honouring while quelling the Blood power of the placenta. In the eastern Woodlands, simple in-ground burials are very common for both sexes of the placenta (Panther-Yates 585). In this instance, the locale of the burial distinguished between Blood and Breath. For instance, Lenape women may bury the female placentae in the lodge, as protection for the lineage women of childbearing age within that lodge (Kraft 29).

Male placentae were likely to receive leaf-and-tree burials or other forms of open-air exposure, as in the "thrown away" but not quite "anywhere" method (Stewart 332). In 1992, the Mohawk poet Maurice Kenny gave an example of such male disposal of a placenta in *Tekonwatonti*—his work about the life of clan mother *Tekonawatonti* (1735-1795), known in English as "Molly Brant." *Tekonawatonti* was the Mohawk wife of the eighteenth-century British "Indian agent," Sir William Johnson, but because there are no written records of a Western-style wedding, European sources wax frothy over calling Johnson her husband, insisting that she was his "mistress" instead (Kidwell 61). This is, however, to privilege European patriarchy in the old colonial way. The fact is that the matriarchal Mohawks did not use the same marriage forms as the British, nor were Indigenous marriages ever made dead bugs on bark—that is, written down, ink on paper, something tradition-ally called "pen-and-ink witchcraft," mainly useful for making a European lie stick (McKee 11). *Tekonawatonti* and Johnson were married, all right, just under Mohawk law, with the marriage every bit as valid as if it had been consummated under British law.

Tekonawatonti lived through the great horrors of the American Revolution, which visited massive misery and death on all Six Nations of the Iroquois in the service of seizing their land for the settlers, post-war (Mann, *George Washington's War* 27-37, 51-

110). *Tekonawatonti* had nine children, although most sources record only the eight who lived (MacLean). Of the stillborn child, Kenny speaks in the voice of *Tekonwatonti* to say "I left my son's placentas in leaves, tied with wild grapevines" (Kenny 157).

Leaf wraps were a Breath-male burial style, and, yes, Kenny has *Tekonawatonti* say "placentas," plural. "Born" after the infant, the placenta is viewed as the infant's twin, illuminating all the twin stories so common to Indigenous America (Hultkrantz; Radin; Gow 107-108, 150). The child's ceremonial naming was sometimes associated with the "death" of this placental twin. The Hopi people of the southwest desert, for instance, kept the placenta for twenty days, until the ceremony in which the infant received her or his name. At that point, the child's deceased "sibling," the placenta, was buried in the ground (Long 237). Thus, both of *Tekonawatonti*'s "children" had died.

Men living in matriarchal cultures have what a fugitive Freudian may call "womb envy." The male sweat lodge is, for instance, a replication of menstruation, a sort of consolation prize for wombless men. This is why, traditionally, men cut themselves to bleed during the sweat, their Blood going to ground as does a woman's menstrual blood (Mann, *Spirits of Blood* 88-89). This is also why among the Utes and Paiutes of the Southern Great Plains when a man's child is born, he must sweat and then throw out his old clothes—that is, shed his placenta, too (Stewart 332). Among Salinan peoples of California, the mother and new infant also sweated, as women do in grief over a death, here, of the placental twin (Kroeber 159).

As the reader may have surmised by now, the umbilical stub was considered part of the placental afterbirth, but it courageously remained behind with the infant to accomplish a special job. As the Iroquois put it, the task was to act as the great connector, the "solid chain" that linked even babies not yet conceived to the eldest of the lineage women (Fenton 41). Thus, do we all link back to *Atensic*, Sky Woman, the First Woman, and her daughter, *Katsitsiaí:ionte*, Hanging Flowers, the Lynx (Mann, *Iroquoian Women* 33). The "connector" idea helps explain why the Utes would pull the placenta out by tugging gently on the umbilicus (Stewart 304). The solid umbilical chain was and remains the

Iroquoian definition of matrilineage. "Chains," which include the idea of "shininess," are always spiritual descriptors for the Iroquois, even when applied to banal political events, such as a chain of friendship (peace treaty).

The portion of the umbilicus still attached to the placenta is treated as part of the placental twin. Western anthropologists recorded that among the great agricultural nations of Turtle Island, the placental umbilicus was buried with the placenta, specifically to connect the child with Mother Earth (Cushing 184). This is another of those times to be wary of the anthropological record, however, for it was primarily women who were spoken of as being Earth connected in this rooted, growing way. Among the Iroquois, for instance, the number of children any women would bear was imagined as squash tubers running from her womb and through her vagina to dangle down between her legs, hugging the ground (Parker 30). Thus, I am pretty certain that the notion of the cord connection to Blood Earth was a record of a women's tradition. Men's cord burials would have gone to a tree burial, as vines hanging from tree limbs are Breath Sky—another reason that *Tekonwatonti* first wrapped her deceased son and his placental twin in leaves.

The umbilicus was cut near the infant's navel by various methods, as appropriately connected with the child's primary cosmic half. The anthropological record is as sloppy in recording these methods as in recording where and how the placenta is disposed of—that is, without regard to the child's proper cosmic interface. Typically, anthropologists just said such things as that the "umbilical cord is cut with stone knife" or with a "sharp cane" (Stewart 306, 332). Stone, especially flint (heavily used for knives), is an earth element so connected with the Blood half that it was used on girls' umbilici, whereas cane, or any stick pertaining to air, is so linked to the Breath half that it was used to cut the boys' umbilici.

Traditions are full of stories, varying by culture, about the proper way to treat the umbilical stump that remains attached to the child, but the method inescapably addressed the child's cosmic interface. Again, this fact is next to impossible to discern from the anthropological record, which presents two or three methods as willy-nilly alternatives. For instance, the desiccated "remnant of cord" is severally recorded for the Utes and Paiutes as having been put in a "rat burrow" or in an "antelope wallow," or as sometimes "buried" in the "birth house" (Stewart 332). There are three distinct purposes at hand here to be sorted out. Rat burrows are Earth/Blood and consequently for females, whereas antelope wallows connect with hunting, which is Sky/Breath and thus for males.

What about the birth-house burials of the Utes and Paiutes? These were female associated and were seen as protection for at-risk mothers. Men were never allowed in a birth hut because the heavy Blood medicine involved in childbirth might kill them. Should a man be involved, it meant that an emergency was at hand with no other women present, like the emergency aid rendered to a pregnant woman alone on a trail with men, as recounted in an eighteenth-century Lenape history (Heckewelder 340). As did the Lenape chief when she suddenly went into labour, emergency-responder men would sit outside the birth hut all night to ward off predators (which smelled the blood) or to provide necessities to the birthing woman by carefully placing them outside the door but within reach of the woman inside. West of the Mississippi River, Cheyenne fathers stacked firewood outside and brought water to the site for use inside the birthing hut (Capps 85). Clearly, then, the cords buried inside birthing huts were female, whereas the cords buried outside it were male, as in the Pueblo practice (Whitman 31). Likewise, the Lenape burial "outside" a birth hut, as mentioned in an ethnological source, almost certainly meant an outside burial of male placentae, for the inside burial was clearly of the female twin (Kraft 29).

There was also a distinction drawn in the way to secure the cut stump. Among the Hopi people, for instance, if the infant were female, then the stump tie was made of vegetal "fiber strings" (Stewart 306), because the females were the farmers, and was secured using a cooking spoon (Parsons 100), because the women cooked the food they grew. The umbilical tie of a boy, meantime, was made of buckskin secured to an arrow stick, as done by the Utes and Paiutes, because deer hide was Breath appropriate to male hunters (Parsons 100; Stewart 306).

The umbilical stump is retained as a spirit shield of the child's health and welfare. As any mother knows, the stump falls off of its own accord within two weeks of birth. At that point, it is traditionally deposited for safekeeping via methods in keeping with the primary cosmic half of the child. By and large, for girls, the cord is placed in a small pouch cut in the shape of a turtle and then elaborately beaded (Taylor 41; Lowenstein and Vitebsky 22). Farther west, lizard pouches do the trick for boys (Ricky 30). Also for boys, the umbilical pouch is sometimes specifically hunt-Breath appropriate, made of squirrel or deer hide. Plains infants were found buried wearing their prairie-dog-skin pouch over their still-attached umbilical stumps (Guernsey and Kidder 13–14, 18, 33, 58, 60).[5] In the southwest, the umbilical pouch is painted bright red (the colour of success) and, if possible, is made "shiny" (Stewart 306). Anything shiny is a spirit portal. Once the child has grown up, the pouch containing the stump is turned over to her or him (Stewart 306).[6] Interestingly, a carved, Woodlands gorget (throat covering) dating to 2,000 BCE displayed a four-legged animal with a fish tail, whose umbilical stump was still attached (Parker and Stanton 443). Despite the great distance in time from the carver, the fish-water association (Blood) used in a gorget smothering the larynx (Breath) most probably represented a female potency of some force and could well have been the prize item in a midwife's bundle.

The association of blood clots with birth also connects with the widespread custom of painting burials with dull red ochre. In recording this much in 1982, historian James Axtell presented the (red ochre=placental blood) equation as a purely scholarly formulation (123). Had he asked any actual Indigenous women, however, he would have discovered that more than indicating just placental blood, the colour of the red ochre embodied lingering, drying placental blood clots. When properly buried, these red-ochre clots led to reincarnation, for a new generation.

Improperly left lying about, however, placental blood clots invited something entirely else. Any portion of the afterbirth—including placentae, blood clots, or umbilici—haphazardly tossed away resulted in a wild child, often a giant. Giants are dangerous and, usually, cannibals (Mann, *Spirits of Blood* 96, 138, 148-149,

151-153, 156-161). Such "Thrownaway Boys" abound in tradition. As such, they are cautionary tales that are necessarily direct
artifacts of matriarchy, for in patriarchal cultures, the cautionary
tales connect instead with male semen, carelessly spilt, and thus
unable to create sons (Rosenfeld 136-138).

One story of the Natchez peoples of the southeastern Woodlands
features two Blood violations resulting in two not-quite-right boys.
First, a clot of placental blood, which has been simply brushed aside
instead of properly buried, becomes a male infant (i.e., a living
"twin"). Fed exclusively on deer meat soup as a precaution, the
Blood-Clot Boy still grows up to be pretty large but withal, safely
hunting and eating deer, not people. This much is manageable, but
equal carelessness with the umbilical stump leads to a problem
child. Because the stump is flung off by a reckless mother who
tired of carrying it about, the stump becomes "Thrownaway," the
"wild boy." Growing into an isolated giant, "Thrownaway" lives
on bugs he found under logs (Swanton 222-223).

Sometimes, a Blood-Clot Boy was deliberately grown to act as
an avenger of the grower against the clan of whoever had foolishly
left the clot lying about. This is the scenario of the Yankton Dakota version of a popular Plain peoples' story "The Badger and the
Bear," here as told by *Zitkala-Sa* ("Gertrude Simmons Bonnin,"
1837-1878). Looking for revenge against a bear for her stingi-
ness in hoarding rather than sharing food, a badger deliberately
absconds with the bear's placental blood to grow a Lakota man
to act against the bear (Zitkala-Sa 71-72; Riggs 95-104; Deloria
113-120). In a Teton Sioux story—similar versions exist among
the Pawnee, Arapaho, Atsina, and Blackfeet—a grandmother
deliberately grabbed up spilled buffalo blood and took it quickly
into her lodge. "I do not know what to make out of this blood,"
the grandmother mused once home, wishing it were "a man,"
and, instantly, it became a man who "grew rapidly" (i.e., a giant
acting on her behalf) (Curtis, *North American Indian* 111). Because buffalo are already Blood, the potency of clot plus buffalo
constituted double-Blood medicine.

Blood-Clot Girls also exist in the eastern Woodlands. For instance, in the story of the fearsome male giant, *Tsukalû* of the
Cherokees, the giant courts a human girl, whose mother is fiercely

resistant to her daughter's marrying a giant. (Giants have a habit of selecting tall human women and, not infrequently, gang raping them, see: Mann, *Native Americans* 163-166; *Spirits of Blood* 147, 158). The mother throws her daughter's miscarriage into the river, meaning that the child would have been female. Knowing this, *Tsukalû* runs to the river and fishes out some of the blood, which becomes first one, and then a second, Blood-Clot Girl, with whom he absconds, taking their mother, for good measure (Mooney, "Myths" 339).

Full-placenta Wild Boys are more dangerous than Blood-Clot Boys (or Girls). In the Cherokee creation story as written up by anthropologist James Mooney (1861-1922), Selu, the Cherokee First Woman, Corn Mother, incorrectly tosses the placental twin of her son into the river, clearly a sex-inappropriate disposal; thus, it grows into *Inăgi-utăséñhĭ* ("Boy Grew up Wild"). Selu's son finds Wild Boy, bringing him home and telling his parents that Wild Boy "came out of the river." Filled with "magical powers," Wild Boy causes no end of trouble. For his grand finale, he kills Selu, whose dying act is to turn herself into sustaining crops, primarily corn (Mooney, "Myths" 242, 244). In the version of this tradition told by Marilou Awiatka (b. 1936, Cherokee), the troublesome twins do not directly murder Selu, but kill her by stealing her medicine (i.e., her knowledge of how to grow corn [Awiatka 12-13]). According to *Ayûñinĭ* ("Swimmer," 1835-1899, Mooney's Eastern-Band Cherokee informant), the *Anisgaya Tsunsdi* or "Two Little Red Men" of the Cherokee creation story, whom Mooney called "The Thunder Boys," are actually the Blood end of medicine, comple- ments of the Breath giants (Mooney, *Swimmer* 24; "Myths" 435, 512; Mann, *Spirits of Blood* 132-187). Traditionally, dwarfs can be every bit as untoward as giants (Mann, *Spirits of Blood* 163-164, 167-169, 176-179).

Male "placental" blood-spot girls are generally more troubled than troubling, as in the Arapaho tradition of "Foot-Stuck Child." Out hunting buffalo, a man scrapes his foot, resulting in a wound that swells massively (that is, his foot becomes pregnant). When the bursa explodes, a drop of blood grows into *Häsixtäcisã*, the Foot-Stuck Child, who is taken in by the male hunting party. Himself Blood, the bull buffalo, *Hixanākä~*, marries her, only to have her flee him. Hiding from *Hixanākä~* in a (Breath) tree with the men (more Breath) is not a good idea for *Häsixtäcisä*, for the mixed medicine makes her spit out Blood, which gives her party away. Eventually, she marries an underground stone (Blood), before ascending to the stars (Breath) with her "fathers" (the hunting party) (Dorsey and Kroeber 153-159). This is a very placental story, typical of a Blood-Clot Girl born of fathers. Their mixed medicine (Breath birth and Blood existence) makes it hard if not impossible for them to marry exogamously, hence the failures of *Häsixtäcisä*'s marriages.

Long-Teeth Boys can also result when the placental matter of male infants is thrown into water. (Weird teeth are a giant trait, see: Mann, *Spirits of Blood* 142). This happens in the Arikara story of "Long Teeth and Drinks Brain Soup." A mother dies in a prairie fire while in labour. In desperation, the father cuts her open to save the child, a boy (Breath), but then he incorrectly throws the afterbirth into a lake, thus sprouting the difficult twin, "Long Teeth." Long Teeth and his brother, Drinks Brain Soup, cause their father endless 911 alerts, which he is able to quell only because he, himself, possesses some fairly powerful Breath medicine that lets him prudently burn up all the holy objects the errant pair steal (Parks 474-484). In the process of behaving badly, the boys kill some holy creatures, bringing down the wrath of some Breath spirits of sky, who attempt to discipline them. The twins quickly turn the tables, however, cutting off the hand of the sky giant, leaving behind the five-star "Hand Constellation" (Lankford 235 endnote 61).

As we have seen, in the matriarchal cultures of Turtle Island, placentae, umbilici, and placental blood clots require very careful handling to ensure the wellbeing of all material existence: the flora, the fauna, the landscape, and the skyscape. Otherwise, unbalanced scofflaws resulting from improperly handled afterbirth can cause no little turmoil. Whereas once Indigenous American women disposed of afterbirth with care as a public health measure, today it is almost impossible for Indigenous women to control the disposal of their afterbirth. Even so, traditional women are now safeguarding their children's future by nabbing the umbilical stump for proper bundling.

ENDNOTES

[1]United States, American Indian Religious Freedom Act of 1978 (PL 95–341, 92 Stat. 469; 42 USC 1996, 95-341; United States, Religion Freedom Restoration Act of 1993 (P. L. 103-141, 107 Stat. 1488, 42 U.S.C. § 2000bb1–bb4).

[2]This is the "Olentangy Caverns," from the U.S. Show Caves Directory, Good Earth Graphics.

[3]It runs from the eldest woman to the umbilical cord of the youngest infant to be.

[4]Hrdlička claims that the stone was to prevent dogs from unearthing and eating the placenta, but the larger spirit purpose, of which he was oblivious, was to reconnect with Mother Earth.

[5]These infants were almost certainly male, although the Guernsey and Kidder did not specify this fact.

[6]This is generally true.

WORKS CITED

Awiatka, Marilou. *Selu: Seeking the Corn Mother's Wisdom.* Fulcrum Publishing, 1993.

Axtell, James. *The European and the Indian: Essays in the Ethnohistory of Colonial North America.* Oxford University Press, 1982.

Capps, Benjamin. *Native Americans of the Old West,* 1973. Time-Life Books, 1995.

Curtis, Edward S. *The Teton Sioux, the Yantonai, the Assiniboin.* 1908. Edited by Frederick Webb Hodge, Johnson Reprint, 1970.

Curtis, Edward S. *Portraits from North American Indian Life.* American Museum of Natural History, Outerbridge & Lazard, distributed by E. P. Dutton Co., 1972.

Cushing, Frank Hamilton. "Remarks on Shamanism." *Proceedings of the American Philosophical Society*, vol. 36, no. 154, January 1897, pp. 183-192.

Dancey, W. S., and Mark F. Seeman. "Rethinking the Cole Complex." *Woodland Period Systematics in the Middle Ohio Valley*, edited by Darlene Applegate and Robert C. Mainfort, Jr., University of Alabama Press, 2005, pp. 138-149.

Deloria, Ella Cara. *Dakota Texts*, edited by G. E. Stechert, vol. 14,

American Ethnological Society Publications 1932, pp. 113-120.

Dorsey, George A. and Alfred Louis Kroeber. "Run-in-Water, Foot-Stuck Child." *Traditions of the Arapaho Collected under the Auspices of the Field Columbian Museum and the American Museum of Natural History*, Field Columbian Museum, Anthropological Series no. 81, vol. 5, 1905, pp. 153-159.

Fenton, William Nelson. *The Great Law and the Longhouse: A Political History of the Iroquois Confederacy.* University of Oklahoma Press, 1998.

Gow, Peter. *An Amazonian Myth and Its History.* Oxford University Press, 2001.

Guernsey, Samuel James, and Alfred Vincent Kidder. *Basket-Maker Caves of Northern Arizona: Report on Explorations 1916–17.* Papers of the Peabody Museum of American Archaeology and Ethnology, vol. 8, no. 2, Peabody Museum, 1921.

Heckewelder, John. *The History, Manners, and Customs of the Indian Nations Who Once Inhabited Pennsylvania and the Neighboring States.* The First American Frontier Series, 1818. 1820; 1876, reprint. Arno Press and *The New York Times*, 1971.

Hrdlička, Aleš. *Physiological and Medical Observations among the Indians of the Southwestern United States and Northern Mexico.* Smithsonian Institution. Bureau of Ethnology, Bulletin No. 34, Washington, D.C., Government Printing Office, 1908.

Hultkrantz, Åke. *The Religions of the American Indians*, 1967. University of California Press, 1980.

Kenny, Maurice. "Flight." *Tekonwatonti/Molly Brant (1735-1795): Poems of War.* 1992. White Pine Press, 2002, pp. 155-158.

Kidwell, Clara Sue. "Indian Women as Cultural Mediators." *Native Women's History in Eastern North America before 1900: A Guide to Research and Writing*, edited by Rebecca Kugel and Lucy Eldersveld Murphy, University of Nebraska Press, 2007, pp. 53–64.

Kraft, Herbert C. "The Women of Lenapehoking." *Women's Project of New Jersey, Inc. Past and Present Lives of New Jersey Women.*1990. Syracuse University Press, 1997, pp. 28-30.

Kroeber, Alfred L. "Phonetic Constituents of the Native Languages of California." *American Archaeology and Ethnology*, vol. 10, no. 1, 18 May 1911, pp. 13-241.

Lankford, George E. *Reachable Stars: Patterns in the Ethnoastronomy of Eastern North America*. University of Alabama Press, 2007.

Long, E. Croft. "The Placenta in Lore and Legend." *Bulletin of the Medical Library Association*, vol. 51, no. 2, May 1963, pp. 233-41.

Lowenstein, Tom, and Piers Vitebsky. *Native American Myths and Beliefs*. Rosen Publishing, 2012.

MacLean, Maggie. "Molly Brant: American Revolution Loyalist." *History of American Women*, 2016, http://www.womenhistoryblog.com/2008/12/molly-brant.html Accessed 16 May 2016.

Mann, Barbara Alice. "Ending the Ban on Indigenous Spiritualities." *The Wiley-Blackwell Companion to Religion and Politics in America*, edited by Barbara McGraw, John Wiley & Sons, Ltd., 2016, pp. 291-304.

Mann, Barbara Alice. *George Washington's War on Native America*. Praeger, 2005.

Mann, Barbara Alice. *Iroquoian Women: The Gantowisas*, Lang, 2000.

Mann, Barbara Alice. *Native Americans, Archaeologists, and the Mounds*. Lang Publishing, 2003.

Mann, Barbara Alice. "Native Americans, Christian Missionaries, and the Politics of the Forced School Movement." *The Wiley-Blackwell Companion to Religion and Politics in America*, edited by Barbara McGraw, John Wiley & Sons, Ltd., 2016, pp. 139-148.

Mann, Barbara Alice. *Spirits of Blood, Spirits of Breath: The Twinned Cosmos of Indigenous America*. Oxford University Press, 2016.

Mann, Barbara A., and Jerry L. Fields. "A Sign in the Sky: Dating the League of the Haudenosaunee." *American Indian Culture and Research Journal*, vol. 21, no. 2, 1997, pp. 105-163.

McKee, Alexander. *Minutes of Debates in Council on the Banks of the Ottawa River (Commonly Called the Miami of the Lake), November, 1791*. William Young Bookseller, 1792.

Mooney, James. "Myths of the Cherokee." *Nineteenth Annual Report of the Bureau of American Ethnology*. Washington, D.C., Government Printing Office, 1902.

Mooney, James. *The Swimmer Manuscript: Sacred Formulas and Medicinal Prescriptions*, edited, revised, and completed by Frans M. Olbrechts, Smithsonian Institution, Bureau of American Ethnology, Bulletin no. 99, Washington, D.C., Government Printing Office, 1932.

Njikam, Margaret O. S. "The Management of Maternal Services in Africa: The Socio-Economic and Cultural Environment." *Contemporary Issues in Maternal Health Care in Africa*, edited by Boniface T. Nasah et al., Harwood Academic Publishers GmbH., 1994, pp. 11-26.

"Olentangy Caverns." *U.S. Show Caves Directory*. Good Earth Graphics, 1996, http://www.goodearthgraphics.com/showcave/oh/olentangy.html. Accessed 12 May 2016.

Panther-Yates, Donald. "Mourning and Burial, Southeast Choctaw." *American Indian Traditions: An Encyclopedia*, edited by Suzanne J. Crawford and Dennis F. Kelley, vol. 1, ABC-CLIO, 2005, pp. 585-588.

Parker, Arthur C. *The Code of Handsome Lake, the Seneca Prophet*. New York State Museum Bulletin 163, Education Department Bulletin 530, 1913, pp. 1-148.

Parker, Janet, and Julie Stanton, editors. *Mythology: Myths, Legends, and Fantasies*. Struik Publishers, 2003.

Parks, Douglas R. *Stičiišáxk Ux* ["Lillian Brave"], "Long Teeth and Drinks Brain Soup." *Traditional Narratives of the Arikara Indians, Stories of Other Narrators: English Translations*, Studies in the Anthropology of North American Indians, vol. 4, University of Nebraska Press, 1991, pp. 474-484; abstract, p. 811.

Parsons, Elsie Clews. "No. 58: Hopi Mothers and Children." *Man: A Monthly Record of Anthropological Science*, vol. 21, no. 7, July 1921, pp. 98-104.

Radin, Paul. *The Religious Experiences of an American Indian*. Rhein-Verlag, 1950.

Riggs, Stephen Return. *Dakota Grammar, Texts, and Ethnography*, Contributions to North American Ethnology, vol. 9, Washington, D.C., Government Printing Office, 1893, pp. 95-104.

Rosenfeld, Jennie. "Talmudic Readings: Toward a Modern Orthodox Sexual Ethic." Dissertation, City University of New York, 2008.

Ricky, Donald. *Indians of Oklahoma: Past and Present,* Somerset Publishers, Inc., 1999.

Stevenson, Matilda Coxe. "The Zuñi Indians: Their Mythology, Esoteric Societies, and Ceremonies." *Twenty-third Annual Report of the American Bureau of Ethnology to the Secretary of the Smithsonian Institution, 1901–1902,* Washington, D.C. Government Printing Office, 1904, pp. 1608.

Stewart, Omer C. *Culture Element Distributions: XVIII, Ute-Southern Paiute.* Anthropological Records 6:4, University of California Press, 1942.

Swanton, John Reed. *Myths and Tales of the Southeastern Indians.* 1929. University of Oklahoma Press, 1995.

Taylor, Colin F. *Native American Myths and Legends.* Salamander Books, 1994.

United States. American Indian Religious Freedom Act. PL 95–341, 92. Stat. 469; 42 USC 1996, 95–341, 1978.

United States. Religion Freedom Restoration Act. P. L. 103–141. 107 Stat. 1488, 42 U.S.C. § 2000bb1–bb4, 1993.

Whitman, William. *The Pueblo Indians of San Ildefonso: A Changing Culture.* Columbia University Press, 1947.

Zitkala-Sa. "The Badger and the Bear." *Old Indian Legends.* Ginn & Company Publishers, Athenaeum Press, 1902, pp. 59-74.

6.
Discourses of Love and Loss

The Placenta at Home

EMILY BURNS

MEDICAL DISCOURSE HAS DOMINATED the discussion of childbirth for decades. The placenta is rarely discussed outside of medical literature, with the exception of protocols for the professional management of the third stage within midwifery and obstetrics. Certainly, in social research, the emphasis is on pregnancy, childbirth (with an emphasis on the first and second stages), and, later, the health of the baby and birthing woman. The placenta has become as much as an "afterthought" as it is considered the "afterbirth."

Elaine Jones and Margarita Kay write that the placenta is treated according to the logic of the dominant cultural system in place. In the West, this cultural system is undoubtedly biomedicine. Developed as a concept and a practice around the turn of the century, biomedicine is defined by Hans Baer as a "medical system based on systematic scientific research controlled experimentation" (4). Rather than focusing on social origins as the cause of disease, biomedicine emphasizes pathogens. According to this logic, the placenta is clinical waste; it is incinerated unless someone requests to take it home and, of course, files the appropriate paperwork. As such, "biomedicine is ethnocentric; not only believing that its ways are the best, but usually unaware that there are other ways of considering a palpable object or process" (Jones and Kay 101). Biomedicine is unique in considering this organ clinical waste. Yet social research abounds with examples of the ways in which various cultures treat this organ, beyond merely seeing it as "waste."

Burial is a particularly salient treatment of the placenta; Japan, for example, has a rich history of placenta burial, dating back as far as 300 CE (Takayama). The Onitsha of southeastern Nigeria bury the placenta with a banana stem, palm, or sage tree, which would be later named after the child and would always belong to him or her. As Helen and Richard Henderson relate, "Onitsha people say that to kill a banana tree is to kill small children" (184). The trees are said to attract the spirits of unborn children to the village. The Indigenous Seri of Mexico bury the placenta with five small plants. Although most adults do not know where they were born, they do know where their placentas are buried (Moser). Burial is also practised throughout Polynesia, and in Tahitian burial practices, the placenta represents the connection between humans, the Earth, plants, and islands (Saura et al.). In Amhara, Ethiopia, placentas are buried either in the home or in the community, symbolizing a connection to place and kin (Hannig).

In some cultures, the placenta symbolizes a lost child. In Merchang, Malaysia, the placenta takes on the status of semihuman, as the older sibling of the new baby, and is buried accordingly (Laderman). The placenta is wrapped in white cloth and buried as a sign of respect. In Guatemala, the placenta is sometimes referred to as the second child, which makes proper disposal important. The placenta is, therefore, burned, and the ashes are buried (Cosminsky).

Not all cultures bury the placenta, however. Other research has shown that some mothers in Egypt request that their husbands throw the placenta to the sea, symbolizing the hope of the continuous flow of the baby's life. Others request that it be fed to dogs, as "the running of the dogs is believed to confer longevity on the newborn child" (Morsy 166).

Rachel Colls and Maria Fannin argue that "the burial of the placenta and umbilical cord demonstrates how the making of persons is an inherently spatial practice—one that connects the child to an imagined future" (1099). These rituals, then, perform the important function of situating the spiritual life of new babies into the broader social and cultural milieu of the communities that will raise them.

Thus, the West's practice of incineration should be understood as part of the West's cultural practice of childbirth, which is also a ritual. Biomedicine and hospital policy have significantly informed this practice. For women who birth at home, a new way of childbirth becomes possible, as women and families navigate this experience without the dominance of the hospital bearing down on their decisions. Biomedicine, it is important to note, is still present in homebirth experiences, but it is not the only model at work. This chapter illustrates that for some women, the placenta is not just "afterbirth" but an integral element of childbearing and early mothering.

In the homebirth narratives of the women I interviewed for my PhD, I found that participants consumed, buried, or did not separate baby and placenta at all; instead, they allowed the cord to dry and come away naturally—a practice known as lotus birth. The placenta, once disconnected from the baby (or not disconnected, in the cases of those practising lotus birth), is considered by participants as rich with spiritual significance, symbolizing the links between the mother and the child and the loss of the connection forged in utero. I argue here that the placenta rituals are a meaningful way for women to engage with their birth experiences, including previous pregnancies and births, and represent a complex combination of love and loss, which often goes hand in hand with childbirth and mothering more generally.

The findings presented in this chapter are derived from my 2010 doctoral research, conducted with fifty-four Australian women who were both pregnant and planning a homebirth, or had had a recent homebirth. Participants were located across the eastern Australian states of Queensland, New South Wales, and Victoria, and were located either in the capital cities of Brisbane, Sydney, and Melbourne, or within one hundred kilometres of these centres. In-depth, face-to-face narrative interviews were conducted with each participant, ranging from between forty-five minutes to two-and-a-half hours. Of the fifty-four participants, fifteen were pregnant and planning a homebirth at the time of our interview. When I asked them about their plans for their placentas, eleven hoped to bury it, two hoped to practice lotus birth, one planned to consume it, and one did not know what she would do. Of the thirty-nine participants who had a homebirth within the past three years, thirty buried the placenta, three practised lotus birth (two of which were later dried and buried, and one was later consumed), three consumed it, two gave it to their midwives, and one could not remember. In these narratives, the placenta was an integral aspect of childbirth and was revered, honoured, and even ceremonialized.

I am not representing these narratives as a generalizable account of homebirth experiences or attitudes, or even as generalizable of the participating women. I have privileged these narratives not only because the placenta is so rarely afforded the attention of social research but also because peripheral experiences of childbirth and mothering are important.

Although I have discussed the treatment of the placenta in these narratives elsewhere (Burns), this chapter focuses on the discourses of love and loss framing these decisions. As noted, participants considered the placenta rich with spiritual significance, as it symbolized both the links between the mother and the child and the loss of the connection forged in utero. Additionally, participants who had hospital birth experiences prior to their homebirth experience often framed their narrative via a discourse of mourning for the previous children's placentas that were discarded at the hospital. The burial of the home-birthed placenta was not only a celebration of the placenta as a life-giving organ and of "putting it back to the earth," but a memorial for previously discarded placentas as well.

As such, I assert that discourses of love and loss are not mutually exclusive. In the excerpts below, love and loss present as a complex interplay between deeply felt gratitude for the placenta and its role in keeping babies alive in utero, and a personal mixture of the sadness felt at the end of the birthing journey, which marks a symbolic shift in the reproductive life of that particular woman.

When I met Dianna, a mother of three, she had recently birthed at home and had two other children, born in a hospital. She told me about the plans she made for the placenta of her home-birthed baby—a burial with a native Australian tree. She said she planted other trees for her other children, but there would only be one with a placenta beneath it. I asked how she felt about this, and she said the following:

[I feel] a little bad actually that I didn't even think to ask for either of them because it only really came up for us when we were planning the homebirth. Actually this time, and as soon as we were planning the homebirth, we knew we'd obviously do something with it. It's a bit sad that there wasn't the same ritual. I mean, we had the tree planting and so there was an element of ritual, but not having those placentas there is a bit of a loss.

In this account, the placenta is not part of the normal hospital experience. Dianna did not even think to ask for it. This situation is slowly starting to change, with hospitals in Australia providing waiver forms for those wanting to take placentas home with them, complete with warnings about safe disposal. Dianna continued talking about the significance of placenta burial for her: "I think it's an extraordinary thing. Your body grows a whole organ that has multiple purposes, incredibly complex functions.... It builds this whole organ and then you expel it. I just think that's just extraordinary. I think it is about a level of respect for your body." The complexity of Dianna's feelings toward the placenta is bound by the experiences of her previous births, and the respect she has for it since afforded the process. This was a recurring theme among women who had had hospital births prior to home births. These narratives often included a sense of loss and regret for what happened in hospital.

Selina had two children when I met her, and was pregnant with her third. She had her first child in a hospital, her second at home, and she was planning another homebirth. She mentioned to me her son was two and a half, and she still had his placenta in the freezer. I asked her why she still had it, and she replied:

I haven't decided what to do with that yet.... I don't think I've done anything with it because I feel bad because I haven't got [my other son's placenta], so I don't know how to deal with that.... I've still got breastmilk from when I pumped with [my first son], from five years ago, in my freezer I can't bring myself to throw out. I don't know. It's just, it's important.

When I asked Selina if she had plans for the placenta of her next baby, she said she would plant it beneath a lemon tree in her backyard but added, " I'll probably feel even more guilt then; I'll have two placentas and not the first one."

For Melody, her fourth child was her only homebirth and the only placenta that she kept. She told me about the significance and symbolism of the placenta for her:

> I wanted to do something because she's my last child. I wanted to have a little bit of a ritual I guess. And I found that when I got to her first birthday, because she was my last child I was getting really weepy—just the thought of never being able to do that again.... She was born upstairs in this house with a view of the garden so it kind of happened [to be buried there]. I guess to me, because I hadn't kept any of the other placentas, it was a bit of a symbol of my childbearing years I guess, saying this is coming to an end and so we plant this tree for [her] first birthday.... The children all helped dig the hole, and we all helped put the tree in and dig it back in and water it, and we had birthday cake outside for [her] and it was just who we are. It's important to me; it was more significant to me than anyone else I guess. So I spent a bit of time just being quiet that day, just thinking about it.

Tara had four children when I met her. Only her fourth was born at home. She told me about the burial of this placenta, beneath a tree in her back yard. I asked her how she felt about having only one placenta buried:

> I feel a bit sad. I think I knew with my first compared with my fourth, you know there are a lot of things.... I would have done differently, so yeah, there's a bit of sadness attached to it ... but [I'm] grateful to have had the experience [the] fourth time around, and it's almost like I'm doing it for all the others as well. I guess the things that I did with them have contributed to who I am now anyway, and they'll be

part of that journey…. So hopefully, my children will take that on board and have at least experienced it, so hopefully they'll make different choices than what I did with their first babies, if they have them.

Cassandra told me about why she chose a lotus birth for her second child, after having a traumatic placenta birth with her first child in the hospital: "I just I couldn't stand the thought of scissors cutting something so beautiful and connecting us, and I felt like there could be grieving from the baby and a grieving from me. But it just felt like it was natural at that stage as it is in motherhood. [There are] lots of stages of letting go." Cassandra recognizes here the grieving process captured by the many stages of "letting go" that mothers and babies/children experience, and for her, the placenta represented one of the first. The recognition of grief here is interesting, as it is the grief of a pregnancy ending. Regardless of the happiness felt for the new baby's arrival, the pregnancy has, nevertheless, ended.

For Freja, the placenta held particularly complex symbolic and material value. When asked what her plans were for her placenta, she said the following:

I'm going to bury it or invite some women that I love and trust and do a ceremony to complete my birthing, like a ritual around ending my birthing journey and completing that. So that I can move on and start the new phase of my life, now that I'm not going to birth any more babies and feed babies, which is quite a hard thing to come to terms with if you love birth like I do. So that's what I'm going to use it for…. It kept my baby alive and me. It allowed that relationship to occur between me, my body, and my baby. I don't know. I just feel a sense of connection to it, like the thought of putting it in a plastic bag right now and throwing it into my wheelie bin is just … and I don't really understand why. It's just a feeling like I just cannot bear that thought. And it's fascinating because I didn't realize how attached I was to my placenta until I came to that feeling. You know, I thought that I cannot throw it away.

I just can't, and I guess that's why so many women have them in their freezers because it just feels dishonourable ... or not respecting it. It was part of us, my body and my baby... It's a ritual. And it's giving it back to the earth you know with my participation, so I feel that's respectful to the process for my baby and for me. It's a life-giving thing, so giving it back to the earth feels symbolic in some way. It sits better inside me, for whatever reason. The thought of garbage trucks rolling around seems wrong, but if I'm taking charge of it and I'm doing it, I guess it's part of the birthing process and part of the whole journey. And I never got to birth my others naturally, which is because I always bleed, so I think some of it has to do with that as well. It's my way of completing it.

There is a clear attachment between what begins as biology and what ends up as a material object to be used, kept, and stored in freezers; it takes on a liminal space between the body and the world. The attachment, exemplified by the stories in this chapter, is complicated, personal, and fraught with emotion. The loss, and sometimes trauma, associated with the lost placenta is epitomized in the ownership and responsibility of the home-birthed placenta, so it represents more than one child's story, and even more than one birth.

Colls and Fannin write that the placenta "creates relationships to others, and makes possible a relation with the body as well as the land that is not about a return to an origin but, rather, about the recognition of a wider ecology of relations of responsibility with and for others" (1099). As the narratives in this chapter illustrate, participants did not express animosity with the hospital about the loss of past placentas but rather recognized that it is an attachment that may only be realized at home—when one has the space to experience childbirth without the hospital bearing down. With that opportunity, new potential for the placenta appears, which ignites the kind of regret that may not have been experienced at the time of previous births.

Regardless of birth setting, Jennifer Hall notes that women use spiritual language when telling birth stories, and as such, birth can represent an important spiritual event in a woman's life, regardless where or how they birth. As such, Elizabeth Jesse and Pamela Reed argue that spirituality "should be considered as important as biophysical and psychosocial correlates and predictors of perinatal health" (740). The ritualizing of the placenta indicates an attachment to pregnancy and childbirth that extends beyond the health of the new baby and into the broader emotional and spiritual shifts in the reproductive life of birthing women.

Homebirth acts as a powerful conceptual space through which to examine the experience of childbirth, without the dominance of medicalization dictating birth practice; moreover, homebirth represents the possibility that medicalization is not the only way women come to know and understand the maternal body, including their placentas. The shift in the politics of power at home is a dynamic reimagining of the relationship between birth, women, and space. Such an imagining leaves open the possibility that childbearing can be not only experienced outside of medicalized hegemony but pedagogically reimagined outside it as well. This pedagogy is enacted via the rituals and ceremonies discussed in this chapter as an alternative system of birth epistemology. By engaging in these rituals, the women in this research participate in a culture of change for childbirth knowledge and practice.

WORKS CITED

Baer, Hans. *Biomedicine and Alternative Healing Systems in America: Issues of Class, Ethnicity, and Gender*. University of Wisconsin Press, 2001.

Burns, Emily. "More than Clinical Waste? Placenta Rituals among Australian Home-Birthing Women." *The Journal of Perinatal Education,* vol. 23, no. 1, 2014, pp. 41-49.

Colls, Rachel, and Maria Fannin. "Placental Surfaces and the Geographies of Bodily Interiors." *Environment and Planning*, vol. 45, no. 5, 2013, pp. 1087-1104.

Cosminsky, Sheila. "Knowledge and Body Concepts of Guatamalan Midwives." *Anthropology of Human Birth*, edited by Margarita A. Kay, F.A. Davis Company, 1982, pp. 233-252.

Hall, Jennifer. "Birth and Spirituality." *Normal Birth: Evidence and Debate*, edited by Soo Downe, Churchill Livingstone, 2004, pp. 47-63.

Hannig, Anita. "Spiritual Border Crossings: Childbirth, Postpartum Seclusion and Religious Alterity in Amhara, Ethiopia." *Africa*, vol. 84, no. 2, 2014, pp. 294-313.

Henderson, Helen, and Richard Henderson. "Traditional Onitsha Ibo Maternity Beliefs and Practices." *Anthropology of Human Birth*, edited by Margarita Artschwager Kay, F.A. Davis Company, 1982, pp. 174-192.

Jesse, D. Elizabeth, and Pamela G. Reed. "Effects of Spirituality and Psychosocial Well Being on Health Risk Behaviors in Appalachian Pregnant Women." *JOGNN Clinical Research,* vol. 33, no. 6, 2004, pp. 739-747.

Jones, Elaine, and Margarita A. Kay. "The Cultural Anthropology of the Placenta." *The Manner Born: Birth Rights in Cross-cultural Perspective*, edited by Laura Dundes, Altamira Press, 2003, pp. 110-116.

Laderman, Carol. "A Baby is Born in Merchang." *Midwifery and the Medicalization of Childbirth: Comparative Perpectives*, edited by Edwin Van Teijlingen et al., Nova Science Publishers, 2004, pp. 235-244.

Morsy, Soheir. "Childbirth in an Egyptial Village." *Anthropology of Human Birth*, edited by Margarita A. Kay, F.A. Davis Company, 1982, pp. 147-174.

Moser, Mary Beck. "Seri: From Conception through Infancy." *Anthropology of Human Birth*, edited by Margarita A Kay, F.A. Favis Company, 1982, pp. 221-232.

Saura, Bruno, et al. "Continuity of Bodies: The Infant's Placenta and the Island's Navel in Eastern Polynesia." *The Journal of Polynesian Society*, vol.111, no. 2, 2002, pp. 127-145.

Takayama, Masaomi. "The Role of the Placenta in Japanese Culture." *Trophoblast Research,* vol. 13, 1999, pp. 1-8.

Artful Pause I

PHOTOGRAPHIC ARTWORK BY
CATHERINE MOELLER AND JODI SELANDER

Planting Our Placenta Tree

CATHERINE MOELLER

AT NINE MONTHS, my baby had insisted on staying in the breech position, and I was told I would have a Caesarian section instead of a homebirth. In my disappointment, I decided to keep two things the way I had planned them: having immediate skin-on-skin contact with breastfeeding for my daughter, and keeping my placenta, even in the clinical hospital environment. Thus, my husband strode out of the operating room with a huge grin carrying my tiny swaddled daughter in one arm and a sterile plastic bag containing my fresh bloody placenta in the other.

Since it was deep winter, we had to put it in the freezer at home. It struck me as being such a powerful thing. I felt the need to do some kind of ceremony or ritual with it, and I had thought that one day my daughter and I might plant a tree and put the placenta in the earth with the root ball to nurture the little tree.

The frozen placenta stayed in our freezer, moving twice with us from home to home and freezer to freezer, occasionally being taken out briefly by someone mistaking it for a roast. Years later, we finally bought a house, and one day, I decided it was the day to buy a baby tree and plant it in our front yard with our placenta. My daughter was six years old by this time and was quite excited by this project.

I removed it from its wintery resting place and ceremoniously put it into a fancy serving bowl to thaw. As it slowly began to soften, the blood began to pool around it, and I marvelled at the rich crimson life-giving force that it still held. I found that I felt great affection towards it—in all of its powerful, meaty, and bloody glory—and had to photograph its beauty. It was part of me and part of my daughter when we were still one, its long thick cord serving as a reminder. It had been the first way I had been able to feed her, and it gave me a little pang of happiness to see it there in its brightly coloured bowl.

We dug a hole in our front yard together, and we ceremoniously poured the placenta onto the earth, trickling a stream of blood after it. We marvelled, we said some words, and placed our Japanese maple on top of it and shovelled in the earth all around it, until it stood securely. The little trees roots untwined and fed on our placenta's life force, and our Japanese maple is a now a happy, healthy tree. My placenta nurturing one more living thing makes me feel satisfied, and we now have a shrine in our front yard of the magnificent day of my daughter's birth, which we can watch thrive as she does.

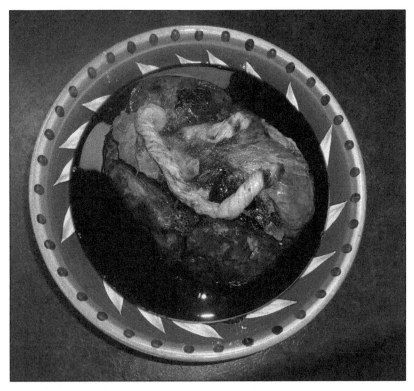

Catherine Moeller, "*Placenta Glory,*" photograph, 2012

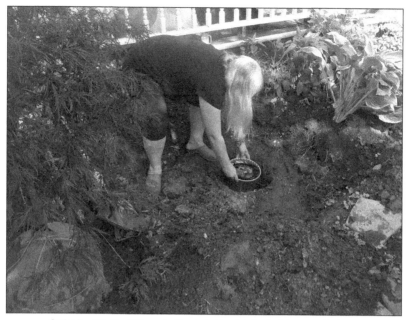

Catherine Moeller, *"Placenta Ready to Nourish Again,"* photograph, 2012

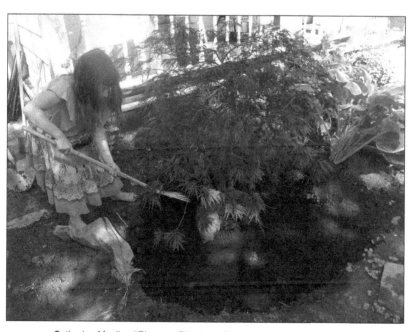

Catherine Moeller, *"Placenta Planting—Sofia's Tree,"* photograph, 2012

Placenta Love

,

JODI SELANDER

JODI SELANDER'S PHOTOGRAPHIC ARTWORKS arose from her understanding of and love for placentas, and aims to capture their beauty. She is the founder and director of Placenta Benefits Ltd., an informational and training organization devoted to human maternal placentophagy. Jodi started researching placentophagy in 2005 during her second pregnancy, and found substantial information documenting its benefits.

Having dealt with depression for many years, Jodi had many risk factors for developing postpartum depression. With a background in psychology, she understood the devastating effects depression could have on women and their families. Jodi found that consuming encapsulated placenta after her daughter's birth relieved her symptoms of depression and gave her additional energy.

As a natural health enthusiast, she launched Placenta Benefits info (PBi) in July 2006 and her initial Placenta Encapsulation Specialist Training Course in 2007. Placenta Benefits has become the world standard in placenta encapsulation training and the only organization with its standard operating procedures on file with the FDA in the U.S., and the FSA in the UK.

More of Jodi's placenta portraits can be viewed at placentalove. com.

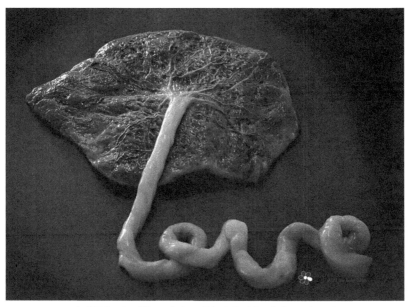

Jodi Selander, "*Placenta Love,*" black & white photograph, n.d.

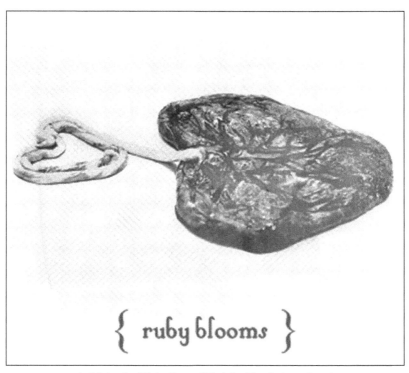

Jodi Selander, "*Ruby Blooms,*" black & white photograph, n.d.

PLACENTERRE II

7.
A Medal for Birth

MOLLY REMER

"CAN I ASK YOU A PERSONAL QUESTION?" asks the woman on the phone. She is calling to inquire about my birth classes, and the subject of homebirth has come up.

"Sure!"

"What about the mess?"

At first, I give the standard answer. That birth isn't so terribly messy, that you can put down towels and chux pads, that the midwife often does the cleanup. I pause a moment. This prospective client and I have an instant connection and excellent rapport.

I add, "Actually, I left a huge blood spot on our living room carpet." I add that the spot came out almost completely with peroxide but can't stop myself from also remarking how I actually "feel kind of proud of it—it felt like a symbol to me." I find myself laughing a little, and there is an unmistakable note of triumph in my voice.

"Of what?" asks the woman.

"That I *did* it. Gave birth in my own home, in my own living room, on my own terms, under my own power, in my own way. In the way that felt best and right and safest to me. On my own. Me. I did it."

What I did not add—what would have been pushing it just a little too far—is that when we moved the peroxide-cleaned carpet square into our new home a large, round, rusty-red stain was revealed on the concrete floor beneath. And that I take secret delight in its presence. I am proud that I left my mark on the floor that bore witness to my labour. I delight and actually revel in the reminder of my power that the stain represents. Is this total weirdness? Or freakishness? A type of maternal masochism or even a perversion? No, I decide. It is really not so different from keeping a football trophy from high school or an award for volunteerism in human services from college. Maybe there is a medal for natural childbirth after all: a blotchy reddish stain on a concrete floor.

Despite our easy camaraderie, I never hear from that prospective client again. Those who critique the zealousness of birth activists sometimes accuse us of supporting an insidious "cult of natural childbirth" and assert that we undermine women and their unique and often traumatic experiences by "insisting" that birth be an empowering and triumphant event for women.

Well, maybe there actually is a cult of natural childbirth, and I am an acolyte of birth, cackling with wild glee as I caper around my bloodstained floor.

PLACENTA RED

I've said for many years that my favourite colour is placenta red—a deep, rich, life-saturated, blood red. I'm amazed by the placenta. How stunning it is that we can grow a whole new organ and then just release it from our bodies when it is no longer needed. The placenta often does not get as much acknowledgment and appreciation as it deserves because it pales in comparison to the miracle of a new person suddenly showing up on the earth as well. Forget growing a new organ, I just gave birth to a new person! So the placenta may be cast aside with hardly a glance or even much thought to its powerful role in pregnancy and the sustaining gift of life it offers.

My first son is born in 2003, and I mean to take his placenta home from the birth centre to plant under a tree. But I forget it, and when I inquire about it during a subsequent postpartum visit, I am told it has been discarded with the "hazardous waste."

My second son is born three years later, and my mom makes a placenta print. The placenta goes into our freezer, where it is excavated two years later. We collapse into laughter as we dig through the freezer for it, my husband saying, "here it is!" To which I respond, "actually, I think that is a squirrel." (*You know you're a redneck if you confuse the squirrel in your freezer with your placenta.*)

My third baby dies during my second trimester of pregnancy in 2009. The placenta does not release until six days following his birth. During this stressful, grief-filled time, I talk to the placenta, telling it I will do something special with it, if only it will please come out. When it is finally gently twisted free by a midwife, it has decomposed enough that it is in many little chunks, connected only by remnants of the amniotic sac. I am so relieved to have it finally gone that I don't care when it is tossed in the trash. Later, I wish I had brought it home to bury and to acknowledge it for having tried so hard to keep my baby alive that it wasn't willing to let go, even after my baby left me.

My only daughter is born in 2011. My postpartum doula is tasked with making a placenta print and encapsulating the placenta. After this birth, I also consume a dime-sized piece of the placenta immediately and feel a huge swell of pride at being "one of those women" who eats placenta. I become a complete fan of placenta encapsulation after this experience and wish I had done so with every birth, perhaps easing the tenuous, tender, exhausting, self-berating months that followed the births of my sons. My babymoon with my daughter is joyous and blissful. My face glows with health, vitality, and exuberance for the first year of her life.

My final baby, another son, is born in 2014. This is my first unexpected pregnancy, and I worry about postpartum depression, so placenta encapsulation is a must. Again, I consume the dime-sized pieces with delight, and I look forward to taking the placenta pills and feeling the same sense of placenta-powered exhilaration I experienced with my daughter. As it turns out, this time I feel headachy, tearful, and "sped up" while taking the pills and happy, joyous, connected and loving without them. I leave the remaining half of the pills in the freezer for menopause instead.

BIRTH ART

My husband and I have a jewelry, sculpture, and pewter casting business. I become obsessed with using one of these remaining placenta capsules to make a jewel to set in the belly of one of our goddess pendants to commemorate this final birth—this final, delightful, most baby of babies.

Why, you may ask? Three possible explanations come to mind:
Why not?
Freaking awesomeness.
Awesome freakishness.
As my oldest son said when he saw us with our placenta powder and our goddess pendant, "Yeah, that's totally normal."

It takes several attempts before we get a result we are happy with. First, we use regular clear casting resin, and it turns out extremely bubbly. The dehydrated placenta "sinks" in the resin and concentrates at the bottom (front) of the mold. The bubbles of this initial attempt make it look "fizzy" and opaque rather than clear and jewel-like. For the second attempt, my husband puts the placenta-filled resin into the vacuum chamber he built, which reduces bubbles. This version does not look cool. It bubbles up in an extremely dramatic way that we've never seen before and creates a weird mutated effect. We hypothesize that the weird bubbling must be a reaction to having organic material in with the resin and almost give up. With a little more research, we decide to give jewelry resin a try instead of the casting resin we've been using. Finally, we have a placenta jewel good enough to set.

I have a favourite quote from Susan Piver that I often share at mother blessings, which are women-centred ceremonies to celebrate and honour birth and mothers-to-be. The quote reads as follows:

> The memory of [my child's] birth has become a talisman that I hold in my heart as I journey deeper and deeper into motherhood. For these moments come again in every mother's life—the times when we are asked to walk straight into our pain and fear, and in doing so, open up to a love that is greater than anything we ever could have imagined: all life's beauty and wonder, as well as all the ways that things can break and go wrong…. Again and again, motherhood demands that we break through our limitations, that we split our hearts open to make room for something that may be more than we thought we could bear. In that sense, the labor with which we give birth is simply a rehearsal for something we mothers must do over and over: turn ourselves inside out, and then let go. *(23)*

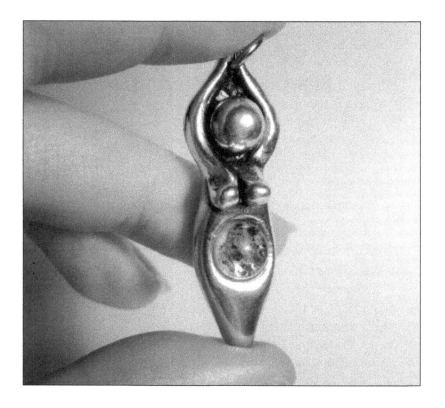

Birth art, birth jewelry, and even bloodstained floors can be tangible "talismans" of our birth journeys. We can draw upon past moments of strength for inspiration and encouragement and affirmation during current struggles. During the day, I often carry around the birth goddess sculpture that I held during my labour with my last baby, and I set her by my bed at night. She reminds me of what I am capable of. My placenta jewel pendant offers the same affirmation and connection.

You know how it is said there is no medal for giving birth?

I disagree.

WORK CITED

Piver, Susan. *Joyful Birth: A Spiritual Path to Motherhood*. Rodale Books, 2002.

8.
Planting Our Placentas

FARAH MAHRUKH COOMI SHROFF

Placenta adentro
Gracias a ti, placenta
My baby is nourished
Gracias a ti, placenta
My baby breathes
Gracias a ti, placenta
My baby releases toxins
Gracias a ti, placenta
My baby is safe from infections
Gracias a ti, placenta
My baby's blood flows
Gracias a ti, placenta
My baby is entering the world

Placenta afuera
Placenta! You're a pillow of life!
Placenta! You're in hands of my midwife
Placenta! You're in a circle of love
Surrounded by Mom, Dad, Baby, and Peace Dove

Flying
        Outside
                We go!

Placenta adentro
Planting you, placenta, under this tree

Implanting you, placenta, deep into a new mother
From inside my womb
                    your new home is this earthly room
You will once again be
Nourisher and nourished, connector of life, past—present
Over tree roots
Joined forever to baby's boots

STORIED PLACENTA NOTES

In Parsi culture, we celebrate fertility with an *agarni* ceremony, in which community members gather together to rejoice in the coming of the new baby at seven months into the pregnancy. We eat special foods, and the expectant mother receives gifts for the baby. My sister and I planted some of the *agarni* foods—rock candy, almonds, coconut—under a sapling that we buried in the forest just after the ceremony.

Once both our babies were born, Roozbeh, my beloved, and I created a placenta ceremony. We hosted a ceremony at home with family and friends. Our babies' adopted Afrikan grandfather came from Toronto to Vancouver to lead us in thanking the ancestors and then burying the placenta under a tree. My sister had found a tree astrology, and Zubin, our eldest, had his placenta buried under a fig tree. Our younger son, Arman, had his placenta buried under a walnut tree. We learned later that this is an ancient tradition from many Afrikan cultures, and being proud to have been born in Kenya, we were carrying this on in our Canadian home. This was a new celebration for our family and our culture—one that we improvised with creativity and love. My Iranian husband and I have enjoyed carving out such new pathways for our kids ever since.

Within a generation, the placenta ceremony has gone through metamorphosis. The only Parsi placenta tradition that I know about is the one that my Grandma performed on me when I was still on the delivery table. My dad tells the story with a great deal of hilarity. As soon as Dr. Ansuya Desai would allow it, Granny picked up the placenta and vigorously rubbed it all over my freshly arrived body. I literally became a bloody mess. Granny and Mom seemed quite pleased that they had performed this rite for the first-born granddaughter. Had I been a boy, it wouldn't have been necessary. From their perspective, they had given me the best chance of growing up with little hair on my arms, legs, face, and other spots. The idea of a smooth skinned, hair-free girl was very appealing.

Now, gazing at the virgin hair on my arms and legs, unshaven mainly because of my early feminist ideals (at age ten, I suggested to my girlfriends that we didn't need to shave our legs if the boys weren't going to do it and I have never done so) I giggle aloud. I don't make a big deal of this. It feels more natural, and as a yoga *sadhaka* (aspirant/practitioner), I have learned that being myself is an important part of this journey. I am not trying to make a big point. However, it's the hair under my arm pits that has created quite the conversation starters. "Why do we need armpit hair?" is usually the way the dialog begins.

9.
Circling the Red Tent

ALISON BASTIEN

Amongst the Seri, an almost-extinct tribe in Northern Mexico, the standard greeting is "*Miixoni quih zo hanta no tiij?*" Literally translated, this means "Where is your placenta buried?" The Seri can indicate the exact spot—covered in desert sand and ash and marked with a ring of stones—where their own placentas are lovingly interred (Rymer). Few of us could respond at all to their greeting. To the Seri, this would be akin to not knowing who you are.

WHERE IS YOUR PLACENTA?

Where is your placenta? For most of us, our placentas were just thrown in the trash. When I was a labour coach in hospitals in California and in Mexico in the 1980s, a plastic slide was attached to the bottom edge of the delivery table so that the placenta would zip right from the mother's body into the trash basket waiting below. Nowadays, placentas are classified as biohazardous waste and incinerated.

Yet the placenta literally anchors us to earthly existence. It insinuates itself into our mother's uterine wall so that we can begin to share our lives. A fully formed and attached placenta signals that the period of greatest danger of miscarriage has passed. The baby sits peacefully by its placenta, not unlike how the Buddha sat by the Bodhi tree, awaiting enlightenment. Ultrasounds reveal that babies like to rest their heads against the placenta in utero, like a pillow pulsing the ocean's lullaby, as they listen to their mother's blood flowing through the cord to them.

PLACENTA MEDICINE

Placenta medicine is now in the media. There are websites, Facebook pages, mainstream magazine articles, and workshops touting the benefits of eating the placenta and of using a professional encapsulator. A disturbing outcome of this, however, is commodification. Now, doulas, midwives, and specialized encapsulators can take away your placenta, *and sell it back to you!*

I understand that a lot of mothers have no interest in processing their placenta, or are already overwhelmed with their newborn. I understand that sometimes it just makes more sense for one of the birth team to prepare the capsules right away. I understand that many hospitals will not let "just anyone" (i.e., the parents) take the placenta from the hospital, so being a certified placental encapsulator who follows local health regulations can be advantageous.

Nevertheless, I am uncomfortable with the new profession of professional placenta encapsulator. Not the women called to do it, but the idea of the profession itself. It worries me, precisely because it does not seem to worry anyone else.

We have fragmented women's experience of childbirth to the point where we now have a dozen experts on board for the modern woman to employ: fertility specialists, prenatal yoga instructors, nutritionists, childbirth educators, prenatal doulas, birth doulas, midwives, the obstetrician, the pediatrician, the postpartum doula, and the lactation specialist. Now add the placenta professional. You may never meet her in person. You can mail your placenta to her or have it picked up. And for a hundred dollars or so, your body can then be returned to you in a pretty jar or box of pills, powders, and tinctures.

This was your body! This is your flesh and blood, literally, turned into a product for you to buy back!

If we believe that women are wise, powerful, and capable and that those women's bodies are designed to bear and birth their offspring safely, then why do we continue to fragment women's experience and our own womanly knowledge into all these specialties? Why do we tell ourselves we need them? Why have we come to this?

I think it's partly because from whichever place on the circle of helpers we stand—be it doctor or lactation specialist or doula—

we are all motivated by a desire to take part in something sacred. Something deep. Something real. Something that affirms our feminine wisdom. Birthing women, newborn babies, and placentas are all part of our great feminine expressions of the divine mysteries of creation.

For hundreds of years prior to hospital birth, all of the functions of these newly mined experts were embodied by one or two midwives attending each woman, and for thousands of years before that by the mothers and neighbours. These neighbour women were called the "God sibs"—the sisters of God (Kitzinger; Davis-Floyd and Sargent; Thomas). They were the women who gathered around, and shared their stories and skills to help each other get through birth. The God sibs morphed over time into the "gossips," and were trivialized by society as ignorant busybodies. But these God sibs were for generations a source of great wisdom and aid within their communities.

The God sibs learned from experience and from each other. They knew what worked and what did not; they knew who was a healing presence and who knew the healing plants. They had each other's back. They did not take the shirt off your back and sell it back to you when you got cold! Not that this is our encapsulators' intent, by any means. Most of them, precisely, intend to share and regain a sense of the sacred with our busy, overwhelmed modern moms. But it misses the mark, somehow.

I propose that we only process a placenta with the actual mother and baby in the room. Often I will have the siblings, spouse, and grandparents in the room as well. Sometimes I invite a mother who has recently given birth to show the new one how. Sometimes I invite a childless woman (often a friend of the mother) to join us to help hold the baby and share in the mystery. The placenta is not made in a vacuum; it is made in the mother's body. It is part of her and her family. A lot of healing occurs when a woman gets to meet with her placenta—especially if she has had a Caesarean or has had a disappointing experience where she did not feel connected or fully honoured. The transformation as she explores her placenta is magical. Family legacies are healed. Self-esteem blossoms. Fears about blood and beauty and worth are reframed. Initially, their noses wrinkle, as women and their partners worry that it is all too "woo woo," even if they approve of the science behind it. But within minutes, a beautiful calm and sense of pride and wonder takes over.

I would love to see women return to the model of the God sibs. You do not need special equipment to make medicine or art from your own placenta. If we, mothers and neighbours, reclaimed our birth rites and just offered to come over and walk each other through this "placenta part," after a while it would not be so hard anymore to find someone who "knew." We would return to our common vocabulary. Kids would think it was normal to have a placenta in the freezer postpartum, possibly their own.

And for those who do not want a placenta in their freezer, then just honour it. The placenta first anchored your child to you. Now you can let it, the cord, or the blood anchor you back to the Great Mother—Mother Earth. Plant something over it. Bury it somewhere on the actual planet where your child can say "I know where my placenta is buried."

DAY OF THE MIDWIFE

One fifth of May, the students from our local midwifery school were celebrating the International Day of the Midwife (as recognized by the International Confederation of Midwives worldwide) in our town in Mexico by setting up a red tent in the local park. We had no mandated agenda; the students themselves wanted to make a presence in the park and invited me to do a ceremony with them. They had hung cloths with red spirals up to enclose and surround a circle of reed mats. An altar had been set up. A dozen or so women sat in circle. I passed around a little watercolour that I had painted of a placenta after a birth; its filmy membranes stretched up around it. Look, I reminded them, we all grew in a sacred and safe little womb tent with red walls. And all of us gathered here in the park today carry our red tent wombs with us, like nomads, all of the time.

Thousands of years before Christ, nomads travelled with actual red tents, which they would set up for the menstruating women, the birthing women; time out of time for those who needed to sit in the centre of their blood mysteries. There were women sharing their menses under the full or new moon, sitting around a fire, sharing their dreams. The red tent literally signaled a place of seclusion and initiation. I talked about how Red Tent groups are popping up in modern societies (Olorenshaw), as women yearn for the community of the sacred feminine. I invited them to consider forming a red tent group, so they could meet each new or full moon, pass the talking stick, and reclaim their experiences of the sacred in their bodies.

We called in the motherline and they recited the following: "I am [they say their name], daughter of [they name their mother], daughter of [they name their grandmother], daughter of [they name their great grandmother], daughter of the earth, sea, and sky, and I am your sister, take my hand." Now holding the hand of the woman next to her, each one recited. We become like the many cells divided at the creation, uniting while at the same time differentiating. Together becoming more.

MOTHERS ON THE MOTHERLINE

Placenta day. Two of the new mothers from the last childbirth preparation class were now eight- and eleven-weeks postpartum and ready to "do their placentas." They arrived with oversized diaper bags and parked their state-of-the-art strollers in front of the house, then deftly popped the canvas-covered seats off the chassis and placed their precious ones on the dining room table. Beautiful new babies snuggled in their nests, with tiny seatbelts fastened.

"My placenta!" Ana proudly plunked a bright yellow plastic bag on the table with a thud.

I picked it up. "You didn't unfreeze it?"

"You didn't say to."

"I sent a message to your phone, this morning, reminding you."

"I never got it."

"It's okay. We can steam yours." I smiled.

Vero pulled out hers in what looked like the same yellow bag. I untied the knot in the top of the bag and realized the black letters are not from some fancy department store. They read: WARNING. BIOHAZARD. HAZARDOUS WASTE. TOXIC.

Vero laughed, turning to Ana, "That's the bag they gave at the clinic, right? I have the same one"

"There are a lot of options for what we can do with your placenta," I began. "You can do as many or few as you like. And over there is the placenta garden, if you prefer to return it to Mother Earth. We can plant a tree or rosebush over it."

I ran through the many things we could do with their placentas: the art print, the medicine, the beauty products, the dried membranes, and the reasons—spiritual, cultural, medical, artistic.

"I want all of it!" Vero surprised me by announcing. She was a nurse from Argentina. I was not sure whether she would warm up to all this.

Ana shrugged and raised one eyebrow. "I definitely want the art print, and maybe the capsules."

While Ana's placenta was placed in the double boiler to steam and thaw, we moved Vero's already thawed out placenta to a ceramic lasagna pan. It was vibrant—as red and bloody as the day it was born. I spread it out so they could take it in. They commented on the size ("Is it big? Is that normal?") and shape ("It's so round!"). I pointed out the maternal side and then flipped it back over to admire "the tree." The veins on this side were thickly raised, a deeper purple-blue, and resembled a mighty oak in the winter. The "trunk" joined the rubbery cream-coloured cord as it trailed off near the bottom.

"The tree of life," I mused. "I think this is where the Biblical stories and the Kabbalah come from. See how the cord looks like the snake or the trunk? This is the creation story right here!" I pulled the amniotic sac up and out with my hands.

"Look! Baby's first house!" I said, and both women sucked in their breath.

"Here you can see the placenta is like a huge mural on the wall of the baby's room. This is the first thing your baby saw, this beautiful tree, making its soothing noise like the waves at the shore."

The membranes I was holding out with my hands were firmly attached around the rim of the placenta, making a perfect thin red bubble. We could see the hole where the baby had exited from the sac. We could see, as though peeking into the cocoon a butterfly has left behind, the cozy expandable orb of this strong yet gauzy tissue.

"Look, Carla!" Vero hastily unbuckled her chubby daughter from the car seat, holding her aloft before the doorway of the cocoon.

"Take a picture! Take a picture!" She tried to place her back inside the orb. The bloody slab resembling meat in my lasagna pan had transformed into a magical bubble with a purple tree inside a red tent.

THE RED TENT!

How I loved the idea of a red tent when I read about it in the novel by Anita Diamant of the same name. And in my studies of the seclusion rituals of menses, I realized women had gone to the red tent not as punishment, or because they were "unclean," but because they had so much power. Women's mysteries were blood mysteries. Women bled with no wound. Women made new humans by holding in their blood. Women turned their own blood into milk. Nomadic women, tribal women, modern women—all were seeking this return to time out of time. As the new mothers and I looked on this glowing red nest, its gossamer walls of the amniotic sac, I realized we all came out of an oasis of sorts; we all came out of a red tent. The amazingness of ordinary life washed over me, as I sought out the little fold over on the edge of the amniotic sac to carefully peel back the chorion from the amnion to show the mothers.

"Look," I said, and they peered over my shoulder with disbelief as if I had pulled a rabbit out of a hat. "See the two layers of the amniotic sac, the baby's side, and the mother's side?"

Concentrating on not ripping the delicate tissue, I cut it away from the placenta and spread it on a piece of wax paper. It looked like a miniature set of angel's wings. I covered it with another sheet of wax paper to dry. Once dried, it would turn into a cream-coloured, paper-thin piece of leather—pliable and strong. I told them how some cultures stretched this dried skin over a drum or created the baby's first rattle with it. Others wrote a special prayer to the baby on it. Ana wondered if she could do this with hers now. But hers was being steamed in the kitchen. It had become a shriveled grey blob, which I placed in a pie pan for her to examine. Ana's face reflected her disappointment. Her birth had been hard, painful, and ended in a Caesarean. Vero's had been short, joyful, and ended in her husband's arms in the hot tub. I wanted very much for Ana not to feel short changed by this experience, but it was already looking that way. So I spread out her tiny placenta to admire the tree.

"Let's read the future a bit, here in the placenta," I suggested. "Here, we have information about the baby's destiny."

We looked at the position of the branches of the tree, the orientation of the trunk, its size and placement, the areas calcified, and the areas strong. We interpreted it much as a psychologist would interpret a drawing in an art therapy class, and we let Ana do most of this herself. Together, the three of us extrapolated metaphorically on Gabriel's spiritual tendencies, his rootedness to this life, and as we went along, I saw the tension melt from Ana's eyebrows. Then they sliced the respective placentas as thinly as possible onto cookie sheets, to cook them into dark, crispy strips, and grinded into a fine powder for the Chinese medicine capsules. These would be useful for creating more breast milk, for combating depression and preventing haemorrhage; they would also be used as immune stimulants, for mother or baby. We made tincture of Vero's blood for later and to make homeopathic pills. The babies slept, woke, nursed, and were changed. The mothers, tired and satisfied, snuggled in their chairs, nursing their little miracles while the placenta pieces cooked. Vero insisted Ana take pictures of her enthusiastically participating in every step of the process, especially sawing away at the raw placenta with both kitchen scissors and steak knife. Ana, not wanting to do any of that part, insisted the smell was making her nauseous and asked me to help out.

"You a vegetarian?" I asked Ana gently. "Me too."

"Me too!" Vero laughed, waving her bloody steak knife for Ana to take yet another picture.

"What kind of Argentinians are you guys?" I teased. "Aren't you from the meat eating capital of Latin America?"

Vero agreed. "My mother said I was an embarrassment. She was always having meaty cookouts, but I just never liked it."

"Me neither," Ana agreed.

The two sat in silence, nursed their babies, and absently stroked their soft hair.

Ana added, "And I always hated tango. It was, like, for old people."

"Exactly!" Vero nodded. "Reminds me of Sundays at my grandparents' house!"

We sat quietly, the strange liver-like smell of the placentas in the oven, the birds singing in the garden, the subtle noise of nursing babies swallowing their milk. After a while, Vero commented that now that she is so far away, the tango does not seem so bad.

Ana said quietly, "Do you think you could teach me a few of the basic moves?"

"Of course," Vero said. They were circling back now to where they came from, their roots in Argentina. They would go home for Christmas, show off their babies, maybe dance a triumphant tango.

We can never return to our little red tents, though, even if we want to. But at least we can know it was there and that we all came from the same place, really.

STUDENTS

Today, I teach the placenta class to the midwifery students. Ten of them are in their second of three years in a government-approved school. Although I will do and say exactly the same things with them as I do with the mothers postpartum, none of it will feel the same. They will leave grateful to me for showing it, and they will admire the placenta as a versatile organ. But they will not look on it with new found propriety. They will not ask me to take pictures of them proudly dangling their babies aloft next to it, as though introducing a new family member. They will not move from slight revulsion to a deep sense of ownership of their own miraculous creation, their own connection from nothing to someone to the earth again. They will have to be aware of the blood-borne illness and hygienic handling in a way that mothers processing their own placentas do not.

Now that I have had ample opportunities to share this exploration with mothers and others, I feel more strongly than ever that this honouring and "processing" of the placenta is something to be done with and by the mother. It is a reclaiming and releasing of another of her creations. It is particularly healing for women

111

who had painful experiences or felt ambivalence about their birth or baby. I teach midwives about the placenta not so they can take this as another professional skillset but as a way to give back to the mothers they serve. And so it went.

The whole class loved using the blood in the lasagna pan to smear on the placenta top and press a clean sheet of paper on to make the artistic print of the tree. They were surprised to see the red tent where the baby had dwelled. When it came time for making the capsules I was unprepared for their curiosity. As I brought out the steamed placenta for them to thinly slice before cooking in the oven, one of the students said softly, "I'd like to taste it." Another said, "Could I maybe have a little ... to eat?" This had never happened in class before. I put out some knives, forks and plates, salt and lemon, and invited whoever wanted to have some. A half-dozen girls gathered and took thoughtful bites. They were not newly postpartum women. This was not even their placenta; it was the placenta of a woman who had given birth peacefully in their clinic tub a few days before. I doubted very much this was part of the school-approved curriculum. But the reverence, the curiosity, even peace, I saw on their faces as they chewed their little bites was something I rarely see in class.

HOLY COMMUNION

Academics call it "placentophagy," this custom of eating one's placenta postpartum. Anthropologists and midwives refer to cultures where this took place and to all the other mammals that eat their afterbirth (Bastien; Enning; Lim). There are articles online about the vitamins, minerals and hormones you get from the placenta, about the whole stem cell issue, and about how all the building blocks to create every other organ and cell in the body can be extrapolated from the placenta (Sanchez Suarez; Selander; Nguyen). In the 1970s, the underground midwifery publications would print recipes for "placenta smoothies," which could be whipped up in the blender so that mothers would recover faster from the birth and create more milk. Midwives nowadays sometimes tuck a little chunk of the raw placenta in a new mother's mouth if she is haemorrhaging postpartum or part of the placenta will not come out.

A while ago, a couple wanted to eat their placenta soon after it was born. The mother had made a minestrone soup base beforehand; it was in a pot on the stove when she went into labour. She instructed me to chop her placenta into bite-sized chunks and to stir fry them, then add them to the soup base and serve it to her after the birth. So I did. I have to admit a part of me admired placentophagy and all its benefits, and another part of me—the vegetarian, I guess—thought the whole thing was a little yucky. But this was not about me, and I was happy to comply with the mother's wishes. When I brought the steaming bowl of minestrone-placenta soup to her in bed after she and the baby were all snuggled in, to my surprise, she first gestured the bowl to her mother, who had flown in from the U.S. to be at the birth.

"Mom? You want to try some?"

Her mother made a face. "Oh honey, I don't think so, really." She demurred, but then, as though perhaps she realized this may be her only chance in life to taste such a thing, she said, "Well, just a bite." And her daughter spooned some into her mother's mouth.

"Mmm," her mother said, surprised.

"Honey?" The new mother gestured to her husband, who made a similar dubious expression before opening his mouth to receive a spoonful.

Their two dogs, which had until now been their children, were served some and lapped it up. The new mother sat back on her bed again and ate her steaming soup with gusto. In the low light of the predawn, with the candles burning in the bedroom, and the family all sitting with blissful looks on their faces, the whole placenta-eating thing changed for me. Suddenly, I thought about church, and how they eat the symbolic flesh and drink the symbolic wine while saying: "This is my body; eat this, and remember me. And this wine is my blood; drink it, and remember." I wondered if long ago this was what Jesus meant by Holy Communion. This family was sharing their flesh and blood, literally, in the soup broth, all of them taking into themselves the creation of a new being in the world, all of them making that baby and that placenta truly a part of their flesh as well. No church had rivaled the blessing and the wonder I felt at witnessing this particular form of Holy Communion. There was only the sound of the baby nursing, tiny little glugging noises, and the occasional happy sighs of the parents and grandparents in the candle glow.

I slipped back into the kitchen and turned off the bubbling soup.

WORKS CITED

Bastien, Alison. "Placental Rituals, Placental Medicine." *Midwifery Today*, vol. 71, 2004, pp. 54-55.

Davis-Floyd, Robbie, and Carolyn F. Sargent, editors. *Childbirth and Authoritative Knowledge*. University of California Press, 1997.

Diamant, Anita. *The Red Tent*. Picador, 1997.

Enning, Cornelia. *Placenta: The Gift of Life*. Motherbaby Press, 1997.

Kitzinger, Sheila. *Birth Crisis*. Routledge, 2006.

Lim, Robin. *Placenta: The Forgotten Chakra*. Half Angel Press, 2010.

Nyguyen, Suzanne. "The Amazing Placenta." *The Atlantic*, 13 Dec. 2013, https://www.theatlantic.com/health/archive/2013/12/the-amazing-placenta/282280/. Accessed 18 Apr. 2017.

Olorenshaw, Vanessa. "The Red Tent Movement." *Huffington Post UK*, 7 Sept. 2015, http://www.huffingtonpost.co.uk/vanessa-olorenshaw/the-red-tent-movement_b_8091348.html. Accessed 18 Apr. 2017.

Rymer, Russ. "Vanishing Voices." *National Geographic*, July 2012, http://ngm.nationalgeographic.com/2012/07/vanishing-languages/rymer-text. Accessed 18 Apr. 2017.

Sanchez Suarez, Sergio "Estudio Bromatologico de la Placenta Humana" *Ob Stare*, vol. 15, 2004, pp. 31-44.

Selander, Jodi. "Human Maternal Placentophagy." *Journal of Ecology of Food and Nutrition*, vol. 52, no. 2, 2013, pp. 93-115.

Thomas, Samuel. "Gossip in Early Modern England," *English Historical Fiction Authors*, 11 Jan. 2012, http://Englishhistory-authors.blogspot. Accessed 18 Apr. 2017.

10.
Hélène Cixous

Matrix Writrix

MARIE-DOMINIQUE GARNIER

PREGNANCY. PLACENTA. PLACENTA PREVIA. Post*p*artum de-*p*ression. Parturition. Pre- and *p*ostnatal. Premature. Painless. What has happened to the semiotic and semantic field of birth-related terms? Where have the *b*'s gone? The *b*'s for birth, for being born, the *b*'s for babies and birthing baths, the synchronous *b*'s that give lullabies their beat and rocking cribs their lilt? The *b*'s as in bearing, as in labour, the *b* in womb and belly? The *b* for beginning and for bringing forth? Instead, an overabundance of *p*-prone, phallic ensign bearers seems to have burdened the graphic and phonetic spectrum of birth giving and motherhood.

As for the term "delivery," found for example in the phrase "delivery unit," it appears to have recently given up on its semantic connections with birth in order to accommodate new meanings pertaining to the commercial lingo of what efficiently "delivers." "Delivery unit" in official use, for example in "the prime minister's delivery unit," referred until recently to a centre of government institution in Great Britain. Abolished in 2010, the now-defunct "D.U." has been replaced by a "performance unit," prefaced with yet another power-related "*p*," which probably aims at the same graphic impact as other terms in a similar phallic vein—from paternity to presidency, priesthood, plutocracy, privilege and premiership. Such idioms, initiated by the plosive consonant that gives them pride of place, contribute to confirm, on a minimal, literal scale, what Luce Irigaray describes in *To Speak Is Never Neutral* and later analyzed in the context of the talking cure: "the unanalyzed functioning of language entertains a power which transcends those who speak and listen" ("L'Ordre Sexuel" 82, translation mine). A phoneme, it seems, can literally blaze a trail in the direction of what is principal, paramount, primordial, portentous, in the direction of what "imports." That phoneme "imports," in more than one sense, both in terms of operating as a promoter of *p*-ridden discourse and as an importing, parasitous presence: a flag, a pennant, a pennon.

But perhaps, after all, language and bodies do interact, not only in speech but at the infra-readable, graphic level of letters or monograms. The *p*-branded bevy of terms pertaining to pregnancy arguably displays the mark or mask of an authoritarian presence intent on imposing or regaining some form of control, even at a minimal, literal scale. Perhaps, after all, body-oriented strands continue to inhabit language and to haunt graphemes as well as phonemes: stray chords or cords linking what is only apparently severed.

The phoneme *b*, a labial, requires the joining of two lips for its utterance. On this simple theoretical basis, as well as on the fact that in French "*lèvres*" translates both lips and labia (minora, majora), Luce Irigaray has based her logic of resistance to the power of "the one," the singular, the phallic, in order to accommodate another vocabulary, summed up, for example, in the title of "To Be Two" and in her dissident style. In her work, Irigaray has repeatedly sought to question the strict separation of the real and the ideal, the bodily and the linguistic, although what she terms linguistic rests on analyses of the spoken rather than written word. In what Irigaray termed the "placental economy" (*Je, Tu, Nous* 40), elaborated partly in dialogue with Hélène Rouch, the placenta was conceived as a fetus-generated "third body"—a space "between-two" introducing the possibility of imagining a nonappropriative relation, an "anexact" form of calculus that complexified and questioned the self-other binary.

In the wake of these cross-disciplinary dialogues between Rouch and Irigaray, philosopher Kelly Oliver has taken up the placental model of relational exchange to develop what she terms "placental ethics," premised on the concept of a "subjectivity without subjects." In her study, the mediating role played by the placenta is therefore approached in composite terms, with the help of compounds—in

terms of "socio-bio, or linguistic-material" (*Subjectivity* 89).
Irigaray's more recent articulation of the placenta as both material
and metaphorical interestingly puts the concept of the placental
to the task of rereading Maurice Merleau-Ponty's unfinished last
work, *The Visible and The Invisible.* In a recent essay, Irigaray
describes the philosopher's relation to the world as that of a subject who considers the world around him as, "a kind of placenta
or construction for mastering the beginning of his life" *(Irigaray:
Teaching* 225). Here, her pairing of the placenta to a "construction
for mastering" brings us back to the sense of an implicit gendering
ingrained in the very term "placenta," as described in the opening
series of *p*-related terms pertaining to birth and birthing.

Following the hypothesis that the term "placenta" is literally
gendered, occupied from the start by a daunting, determining
initial, and that it operates, furthermore, as an abstracted, medicalized, Greek-enhanced masculine manifesto disconnected from
the term's initial matter-of-factness —in other words from the term
"ϖλαϰοῦς" or "plakous," a flat bread similar to a layered pie or
baklava—the phrase "placental economy" contains, one could
argue, an internal contradiction: it attempts to gesture toward a
new model of exchange based on bodily limitrophy, poised on the
"anexact" arithmetic of the "between-two," while resorting to a
"masculine" term of control—to the placental "powerhouse."

This essay attempts to trace possible lines of resistance and
addresses the question of how to do or undo things with words.
How can one displace or annul logocentric traces of mastery in
a discourse that seeks nonappropriative paths and new linguistic
and corporeal neighbourhoods? How can literature rather than
discourse or "speech" refashion or explore ways of phrasing things
"placental" in a nondivisive, nonbinary language?

My intention here is to shift focus away from the verbal or
the spoken in order to (partially) analyze some of the lines of
resistance at work in the written corpus of Hélène Cixous, whose
fiction hinges on a nonbinary, complex way of counting: "all is
two, all is minus two all is plus two" (*OR, Les Lettres* 28-29,
translation mine).[1] What if the critical, vital function of literature,
or *"litterature,"* with two *t*'s in French, was precisely to question
the status of "litter," the status of what comes out second of a

birthing body, of the so-called adnexa or secundine expulsed from a body of the "second" sex, annexed to the first? What if literature belonged precisely with the strange temporality of the afterbirth, creatively understood as the ability to be born more than once, in a nonsequential sequence of writing? What if the "placenta" was a blueprint or the marker of an empty place for other names to step in? What are the substitute names and multiple renamings of the "placental"?

What follows begins by exploring the conspicuous absence or suppression of the term "placenta" in a selection of Cixous's writings pertaining to birth (from "The Laugh of The Medusa" to *The Day I Wasn't There* and *Homère est Morte*), before addressing some of its fertile resurgences, substitutes, or replacements—literary and literal avatars of a lost viscus: "manna," "naphta," and what I tentatively call the *"place-en-terre."* Or, in a tentative translation, "earth-birth": a feminized afterbirth or rebirth of the "placental," newly replanted, regrown in a vegetalized form.

BIRTHINGS

Of the same generation as Luce Irigaray, Hélène Cixous has devoted most of her fiction, plays and essays to ways of challenging and addressing what Jacques Derrida conceptualized as the "phallogocentric"—the complex and complicitous assemblage of hegemonic forces voiced in the logos of classic thinking and oppositional metaphysics. Birth giving is one of the prominent and recurrent themes in Cixous's writing, whose mother Eve ran a maternity clinic in Algiers:

> I give birth. I enjoy giving births. I enjoyed birthings—my mother is a midwife—I've always taken pleasure in watching a woman give birth. Giving birth "well" ... Giving birth as one swims, exploiting the resistance of the flesh, of the sea, the work of the breath in which the notion of "mastery" is annulled, body after her own body, the woman follows herself, meets herself, marries herself.... It was in watching them giving birth (to themselves) that I learned to love women ... And in the wake of the child, a squall of

Breath! A longing for text! Confusion! What's come over her? A child! Paper! Intoxications! I'm brimming over. My breasts are overflowing! Milk. Ink. (*Coming to* 30-31)

The child, hardly born, belongs to the same proliferative economy as writing—a vicinity aptly rendered in French by the possible homophony between "*lait*" ("milk") and "*lettre*" ("letter," "literature"). What follows up on the immediate appearance of the child is paper, not placenta—a fluid, staccato outburst of language desperately looking for pages on which to couch a rapid flow of exclamatives. Fluid rather than solid matter is brought to the foreground, together with apparently negative terms ("confusion," "intoxication"), which blur the contours between subjects. A birthing is, in more than one sense, a "giving birth," understood in more than one way. Birth is itself a giving, in the sense that the baby gives birth to writing, as well as to its/his/her mother.

The topic of birth returns to haunt Cixous's malleable, fluctile writing, notably in *The Day I Was Not There*, which narrates the birth of the narrator/author's "Mongolian" child George ("Mongolian" now called Down syndrome)—as well as the concomitant suspension of writing until after the child's death. In the more recent, as yet untranslated *Homère est morte*,[2] the last days and minutes of Eve, Cixous's mother, are recounted as a somber parallel to her own notebook, whose pages on "painless birth giving" excerpted from her 1962 diary of a midwife are inserted in the book's opening leaves. The delivery procedure becomes indelibly joined to the "deadly pregnancy" (32)[3] described, and yet not described, in Hélène Cixous's own, and yet disowned, pages. No placenta there. A sex change as well as a reversal of roles affect the narrator seen through Eve's eyes: "I am her paternal mother" (9).[4] It is Eve's earlier notebooks, however, that provide the initial force field of the book—forming a placental "diary," a diary for dying as well as being born, all in one.

In the bilingual edition of Hélène Cixous's own *Notebooks*, which contain handwritten notes belonging to the author's pre-rough draft stages of writing, the term "placenta" is used once, in relation to a precipitous cutting of the cord by an idiotic doctor.

The word appears in a critical postnatal assessment by Cixous's mother, rendered in the abbreviated style of a notebook:

Il t'a déchiré il n'a pas remarqué
Il a sorti le placenta tt de suite
Ss attendre qu'il soit sorti et il a laissé 1 morceau dedans

He tore you he didn't notice
He took the placenta out straight
Without waiting for it to come out and he left a bit inside.
(*Notebooks* 81)

In the French version, it is important to notice, incidentally, that "*il t'a déchiré*," ("he tore you") contains a typo, a missing "*e*," implying that the "torn" mother is couched in the masculine (the correct feminine version being "*il t'a déchirée*"). In Cixous's *The Day I Wasn't There*, the notebook material returns, incorporated in the narrative and poetic flow. But this time it is attached to the birth of the "Mongolian" child, not to the "delivery of Pif," short for Pierre François, to whom the excerpt is incorrectly referenced by the editor of the Cixous's *Notebooks*[5]:

Georges nous appelons l'enfant. En vérité c'est l'enfant même, la cause des passions. Une lenfance *nous prend l'utérus du coeur, elle s'attache par ses faibles ventouses à la paroi du ventricule. On ne doit pas larguer le mongolien tant qu'il ne s'est pas décollé lui-même, sinon l'on arrache en même temps une parcelle de coeur et l'on risque de laisser un morceau de placenta dans l'utérus.* (*Le Jour* 97, my emphasis)

George we call him the child. In truth it is the child itself, the cause of our passions. A childhood has us by the uterus of the heart, it grips the walls of the ventricle with its weak suction cups. One must not cast off the mongolian so long as he has not come unstuck by himself, otherwise part of the heart comes off with him and one risks leaving a bit of placenta in the uterus. (*The Day I Wasn't* 53)

A "mongolian" child must be allowed time, time to become unstuck like a placenta, Cixous writes. Like a properly managed placenta, given enough time to come out by itself, the "mongolian" child must, uncouthly, be given the time to return and to haunt writing, the time to produce a novel form of writing able to incorporate improper form, bodily failures, and mishaps. Language is literally affected by the child, for example in Cixous's untranslated nonce word "une *lenfance*" ("a ninfancy"), in which article and noun are stuck, ill-detached as in the case of the torn piece of placenta sticking to the uterus membrane. Contrary to the context of the excerpt quoted from the *Notebooks,* the child here is George, not "Pif"—as if, indeed, a generic child or "ninfant" threatened to blur divisions between all children. The word "placenta" occurs in the fiction as what seems to be a direct quotation from Eve's diary, except that, in its fictionally recycled form, it has been displaced, rendered mobile, turned into a substitute for the "mongolian" child and its expected detachability.

Earlier in the same book, the narrator mentions what she calls the "nostalgia for the placental time," after she witnesses the decaying baby's body "dangling by needles to the drip" as a consequence of a feeding anomaly. Her "nostalgia for the placental time when without blows and wounds we were one and the same blood" (35), however, constitutes, as it were, a new anomaly: something, yet once more, in this new occurrence of the placental, "sticks," is not quite right, and manifests a case of nondetachment. First, mother and child are not, medically speaking, "one and the same blood." In other words, the placental "sticks," and is responsible for textual anomalies, for confusion and trouble.

Such is the case, also, in *Les Rêveries de la femme sauvage*, in which the character Eve Cixous brings in, in the final pages of the book, a "terrible thing, which is the *placenta previa* ... you have an obstruction, the placenta in front of the head, like a door" (164, translation mine). The book ends with a scene of a failed homecoming, when the narrator finds herself in front of a closed gate on a white wall—a metaphorical moment of "placenta previa." This is another traumatic scene in which the narrative voice returns with insistence—as if exiting the narrative and being born were one and the same difficult thing: "there is an obstruction over my head, I thought" (166, translation mine). Again, the placenta intervenes in a pathological way, as an obstacle to proper exiting, rather than as a nourishing interface between two bodies. The placental is in need of displacement, rivaled by the sense of a new "place" to be accessed. Its possibly pathological presence may be an obstacle to the fluid remapping of a woman's body, as described in "The Laugh of the Medusa" manifesto, where a woman is, Cixous notes, "body without end, without appendage, without principal parts" (889). It is a text that one could read, yet again, as Cixous's effort to resist *p*-initialed, phallic terms—to fend off, in other words, the language of a medicalized mapping of bodies.

In order to write what she re-envisions as a body without end, as a dissident "matrix," Hélène Cixous, "writix" of many births including her own, must produce an unheard-of style. She must grapple with bodies of plosives and remove "principal parts;" she must invent open-ended terms and lexical junctures for bodies without end. "Manna" and "naphta," explored below, are part of this newly evolved language of birthing. Manna in particular operates both as a nutrition-related term and, in French, as a multigendered noun able to turn "man" into a strangely feminine-sounding term, equipped with an appendixed, feminizing a-ending.

MANNA

In *Manna To The Mandelstams To The Mandelas*, the term "placenta" appears twice, each time in a nonhuman context, bearing no relation to the field of obstetrics. It appears briefly as a "celestial placenta," a phrase aiming to refer to a felicitous, prelapsarian moment in the lives of Ossip Mandelstam and Akhmatova, two of the poets inhabiting this book:

> *A vingt ans on a vu le pont entre les deux parties du monde, l'entrée de la terre encore vierge d'humanité, et l'unique cordon qui unit le Bien et le Mal au même placenta céleste.* (*MANNE* 148)

At twenty we saw the bridge between the world's two parts,

the entryway of the earth still virgin with humanity, and the single cord uniting Good and Evil to the same celestial placenta. (*Manna* 108)

Its second appearance takes place in a birthing scene, whose only redeeming features imply a becoming-vegetal. The fictional voice of Winnie Mandela mourns her lost "man," her lost manna, in a negative celebration of her absent, lacking lover:

J'ai tout ce que je n'ai pas, le manque célèbre en moi les indicibles extases de satisfaction, j'ai sur mes seins tes invisibles et lourdes mains, je suis un amandier qui brûle sans relâche comme deux damnés étroitement mêlés depuis des milieux d'années, j'aspire l'éternité par mes racines aux doigts agrippés, en haut je pars en fumée, sous terre je nais je tète je m'accroche immortellement, je suis plantée de toutes mes fibres moi qui suis redoublée de toi, dans l'utérus du futur.

Le martyre est mon placenta. L'atroce pain. (MANNE 325)

I have everything I do not have, lack celebrates in me the inexpressible ecstasies of satisfaction, I have your invisible and heavy hands upon my breasts, I am an almond tree that burns without rest, like two damned people bound for thousands of years, I inhale eternity through my roots with clutching fingers, up above I disappear in smoke, under the earth I am born I suck I cling immortally, I am firmly planted with all my fibers, I who am doubled by you, in the uterus of the future.

Martyrdom is my placenta. The atrocious bread.

In the bitter kernel the milk seed. The almond is there, in the bitterness. It is the secret Mandela: the manna. The manna come from the heaven hidden under the earth. It has the taste of certainty. Amandla! (*Manna, Cixous Reader* 178-179)

The French version of the text plays on the homophony between the name of the almond nut ("*amande*" in French) and the proper name Mandela, as well as on the German term "*Mandel*" for almond, in pages dedicated to the Russian poet Ossip Mandelstam, celebrated together with the Mandela pair in this complexly woven, echoic text. Man and wife are "like" two kernels, two almonds in the same shell. The severed "almond pair" is revived and re-membered in the textual voice of Winnie Mandela. The double kernel is not unlike the double fruit or "*Obst*" in German, formed by the baby-placenta pair—a term that Cixous plays on in connection with obstetrics (Cixous, *Illa* 194-195). In the beginning was number two. Such is the new, unattested gospel found in *Manna*, a word whose feminine ending, whether in English or in French ("*Manne*"), seems to bear, like a kernel, the seed or syllable of "man." The placenta occurs, here, in the negative context of a "martyrdom," an image that quickly gives way to another, nonorganic semantic field, in which the "atrocious bread" is displaced and is replaced by a vegetal image: kernel and seed. Milk and its "ink" have replaced and displaced the placental metaphor. This milk, furthermore, is not human but vegetal, almond milk—a posthuman transition to what the text calls "manna." This manna should not be mistaken for a godsend, however: the heaven it is associated with is "hidden under the earth." *Manna* introduces, in other words, the language of vegetal, nonhuman, immanent life resources, which should not be severed from what Cixous calls "earth," or "*la terre*."

Earth appears as a constant theme and poetic resource in Cixous's writing. It is also from intimate connections to earth that the non-organic body of Cixous's "Medusa" derives her writerly energies and nutrients. In Cixous's manifesto, substitute terms are yet again used in lieu of nourishing bodily organs. The "Medusa" contains no "placenta," although many birthing moments contribute to its poetic texture as well as to its economy of giving and giving birth. The manifesto refuses to speak the language of anatomized, medicalized bodies. It prefers to lend an ear to "the resonance of fore-language" and to "let the other language speak—the language of 1,000 tongues which knows neither enclosure nor death" (889). The "*I*" has become in this text "more or less human." Earth, soil, and subsoil displace and replace medical anatomies of the body.

NAPHTHA

The text of Cixous's inaugural essay *Laugh of the Medusa* displaces birth-related vocabulary in order to make room for a more fluid, non-organic remapping of bodies. Her style is in search of unheard-of, novel terms, such as the rare, foreign-sounding "naphtha": "Write yourself. Your body must be heard. Only then will the immense resources of the unconscious spring forth. Our naphtha will spread, throughout the world, without dollars—black or gold—non-assessed values that will change the rules of the old game" (880). "Naphtha" refers to the inflammable volatile liquid exuding from the earth in some parts of the world (such as Algeria); it is a constituent of asphalt and bitumen, now used for such products as crude oil or refined products like kerosene. The word, gendered in the feminine in French, is of uncertain etymology—"Egyptian" according to Emile Littré, possibly of "oriental origin" according to the *Oxford English Dictionary*. Naphtha, not unlike manna, oozes through the earth surface—as well as, literally, through the complex surface of its doubled graphic filter of consonants (*ph/th*). Through the uncouth, poetic arabesques of the word "naphtha," Cixous's writing pushes the limits of the organic body and connects it to an outlandish, living expanse of land, whose exact boundaries remain unknown. This time, the Cixousian matrix relies on a non-Latinate term: like manna, based on the ancient Egyptian word "*mannu*," naphtha modifies the map to incorporate non-Western borderlands. Such a body feeds on a "place" without place-markers, without partitionings:

> Women must write through their bodies, they must invent the impregnable language that will wreck partitions, classes, and rhetorics, regulations and codes, they must submerge, cut through.... (886)

In Cixous's manifesto, the "umbilical cord" does not gesture toward maternal connectedness but signals male writing and male syntax—the well-structured line, the well-oiled hierarchy of clauses:

> Such is the strength of women that, sweeping away syntax,

breaking that famous thread, (just a tiny little thread, they
say), which acts for men as a surrogate umbilical cord,
assuring them—otherwise they couldn't come—that the
old lady is always right behind them, watching them make
phallus, women will go right up to the impossible. (886)

In 2012, the umbilical cord returns in a book Cixous devoted to
the painter Pierre Alechinsky, *Le Voyage de la Racine Alechinsky*.
It returns this time in the form of a severed, travelling root or
segmented bamboo shoot: "one must cultivate one's root—both
severed and saved" (16). She adds the following:

> *Il faut dire qu'il n'y a pas plus nourrissant pour l'imagina-*
> *tion que cette espèce d'amphibie végétal, cette tige-racine*
> *souterrienne qui pousse des bourgeons au dehors et émet des*
> *racines adventives dans sa partie inférieure vers le dedans.*
> *De même que le Rêve, nous murmure Freud en sa transe*
> *apocalyptique, est une sorte de champignon qui, au lieu de*
> *racine, pour racine, dispose d'un thalle aux innombrables*
> *nervures subtiles nouées autour de son col.* (17)

Indeed, there is nothing more nourishing for the imagination
than this sort of amphibious vegetation, this underground
root-stalk which grows shoots on the *outside* and sends
adventitious shoots towards the *inside* in its lower half. Just
like a Dream, as Freud whispers to us in an apocalyptic
trance, is a sort of mushroom which, in lieu of a root, by
way of a root, possesses a thallus with innumerable subtle
ribs knotted around its volva. (16-17, translation mine)

What nourishes, here, follows a vegetal track, which Cixous's
writing mimics by producing branching out terms (a "root-stalk")
and rhizoming, composite adjectives— such as *"souterrien,"* a
nonce word that telescopes *"rien"* ("nothing") and *"souterrain"*
("subterraneous") in a portmanteau formation, while recalling the
title of one of Alechinsky's texts (*Rein, Comme si de Rien*). The
placentary or nourishing element has now become what could be
termed the *"placenterre"* in an effort to unite the placental and the

terrestrial, in other words to reconstruct a path between "earth" and "birth." A female-cum-fungal body emerges in Cixous's writing: a "thallus" has, this time, displaced the language of the "phallus," of logocentrism, whereas, on the other hand, a strangely human and vegetal body looms forth in what has now metamorphosed into a quasi-vulvic "volva" or "col," in French—a cervix.

BEVIES

By way of concluding this nonexhaustive study of the poetic and philosophical uses of the placental in a selection of Hélène Cixous's works, one might follow a quasi-circular or spiraling path—a path bringing us back, literally, to the *b*-borne soundtrack of birthing. In "The Laugh of the Medusa," readers are invited to experience a succession of birthing moments, building momentum thanks to the bevy of *b*'s disseminated on the literal surface of this portable, mobile, and nourishing "placental" book: "we the labyrinths, the ladders, the trampled spaces, the bevies—we are black and we are beautiful ... our blood flows and we extend ourselves without ever reaching an end" (878).

ENDNOTES

[1] Translation is mine from the French, "*Tout est deux, tout est moins deux tout est plus deux, tout témoin des deux mondes.*"

[2] The title puns on Homer and "*homme-mère*" (man-mother). A tentative translation for this escaping, restless title could be: *Homère Has Died.*

[3] "*Grossesse mortelle*" is the French, p. 32. "*Accouchement sans douleurs*" is the title of Eve's *Notebook*, p. 14.

[4] Translation is mine from the French, "*Je suis son père maternel.*"

[5] In her commentary of the same excerpt in *Joyful Babel*, Susan Sellers misses the point that the "*accouchement de Pif,*" ("Pif's delivery") in the original notebook, cannot apply to the birth of George. Pif nicknames the narrator's second son Pierre-François. The footnote referencing *The Day I Wasn't Born* is particularly misleading: "the idea of a piece of the placenta being left inside the mother's body is woven into the author's reflection on the legacy

left her by the baby" (27; see also footnote 8, p. 37). The editor of the *Notebooks* misses yet another point by adding that Pif is "the name of a cartoon character" (footnote 1, p. 81)—which is of little use here and adds a source of confusion.

WORKS CITED

Alechinsky, Pierre. *Rein, Comme si de Rien*. Fata Morgana, 2009.
Cixous, Hélène. "The Laugh of the Medusa." Translated by K. Cohen, *Signs*, vol. 1, no. 4, 1976, pp. 875-893.
Cixous, Hélène. *Illa*. Des femmes, 1980.
Cixous, Hélène. *MANNE aux Mandelstams aux Mandelas*. Des femmes, 1988.
Cixous, Hélène. *"Coming To Writing" and Other Essays*. Translated by Sarah Cornell et al., Harvard University Press, 1991.
Cixous, Hélène. *Manna to the Mandelstams to the Mandelas*. Translated by Catherine A. F. MacGillivray, University of Minnesota Press, 1994.
Cixous, Hélène. "Manna to the Mandelstams to the Mandelas." *The Hélène Cixous Reader*, edited by Susan Sellers. Routledge, 1994, pp. 163-179.
Cixous, Hélène. *OR, les Lettres de mon Père*. Des femmes, 1997.
Cixous, Hélène. *Le Jour où Je n'étais pas Là*. Galilée, 2000.
Cixous, Hélène. *Les Rêveries de la Femme Sauvage. Scènes Primitives*. Galilée, 2000.
Cixous, Hélène. *The Writing Notebooks of Hélène Cixous*. Edited and translated by Susan Sellers, Continuum, 2004.
Cixous, Hélène. *The Day I Wasn't There*. Translated by Beverley B. Brahic, Northwestern University Press, 2006.
Cixous, Hélène. *Le Voyage de la Racine Alechinsky*. Galilée, 2012.
Diaz-Docaretz, Myriam, and Marta Segarra, editors. *Joyful Babel: Translating Hélène Cixous*. Rodopi, 2004.
Irigaray, Luce. "L'Ordre Sexuel du Discours." *Langages*, vol. 21, no. 85, 1987, pp. 81-123.
Irigaray, Luce. *Je, Tu, Nous*. Routledge, 1993.
Irigaray, Luce. *To Speak Is Never Neutral*. Routledge, 2002.
Irigaray, Luce, and Mary Green, editors. *Luce Irigaray: Teaching*. Continuum, 2008.

Oliver, Kelly. *Subjectivity without Subjects: From Abject Fathers to Desiring Mothers*. Rowman & Littlefield, 1998.

Rouch, Hélène. "Le Placenta Comme Tiers." *Langages*, vol. 85, 1987, pp. 71-79.

Sellers, Susan, editor. *The Hélène Cixous Reader*. Routledge, 1994.

Sellers, Susan, editor. *The Writing Notebooks of Hélène Cixous*, translated by Susan Sellers, Continuum, 2004.

11.
The Amazing Placenta

The Placenta's Behavioural and Structural Peculiarities

AMYEL GARNAOUI

I TRAINED AS MIDWIFE IN ITALY, after working as an art historian. I was deeply drawn to change my career and support women this way in order to cherish the wonders of our bodies that can create and give birth to new life. During midwifery studies, I was encouraged to discover many things about the amazing placenta. New discoveries are coming from scientific research that are of interest to all who experience, study, and work with pregnancy and birth.

My chapter draws from research I undertook for my graduating thesis in midwifery, in which I focused on detailed scientific studies of the placenta. I will use scientific terminology throughout. But I hope that my explanations of how, why, when, and where the amazing placenta is at work at the beginnings of human life will fascinate all readers, and show the importance of this little known and often misunderstood organ.

I open with scientific inquiry into the placenta's development and morphology, its growth and structure. I then explore the practice of early umbilical cord clamping and cutting, and discuss how this procedure hurts the health of mother and infant. I also look at how the placenta and the mother's brain communicate as well as the role of the father's genetics in fetal development. I end my chapter by exploring "placentophagy"—the practice of eating the placenta—as part of the evolutionary behaviour of mammals. I hope to give the reader insights into the wonders of this intelligent and generous organ, which is capable of accomplishing so many different things.

PLACENTA STRUCTURE AND DEVEPLOPMENT

The placenta is in direct contact with the mother's body and tissues, and not the baby/fetus. How the mother's body "sees" her placenta, rather than her baby, determines the outcome of her pregnancy. The placenta follows a totally different developmental course than that of the baby. Four days after fertilization of the ovum by the sperm cell, the "blastocyst," which at this stage is made of almost fifty-five cells, reaches the inside of the mother's womb, or uterine cavity. The blastocyst has two different types of cell populations: five of these cells represent the inner cell mass (what will become the baby), and fifty remaining cells will produce the placenta. Thus, creating the placenta is a more critical event than designing the embryo itself.

This autonomous development of the placenta holds the key to a successful pregnancy. From the histological point of view, this organ has unique features that no other human organ has. The outer component of placenta's villi, the "syncytiotrophoblast," which is the first tissue that penetrates into the mother's uterus, is very special. It actually looks and behaves like a virus or cancer in the body. As modern evolutionary theories state, the origin of the placenta is due to the integration, sixty million years ago, of viral genomes into mammals' genomes (Ryan). Five percent of our genome is made of retrovirus genes. These have progressively lost their pathogen (disease) power and are responsible for the typical cellular indifferentiation of the syncytiotrophoblast, which is a very unique tissue with multiple nuclei but no intercellular boundaries (*syncytium*). No other cell in the human body exists as a syncytium.

Syncytiotrophoblast shares with malignant tumours the three cardinal signs of the latter: cells of irregular shapes, invasiveness (as cancer, trophoblast is highly invasive), and metastases. In every normal pregnancy, trophoblast cells constantly break off from the placenta, enter the mother's bloodstream, and are carried off to lodge in her lungs. The lungs of pregnant women contain fragments of trophoblast, known as *syncytial sprouts*. They remain there for a while, and then disappear. This trophoblast invasion occurs only in humans and is not seen in higher primates. The remarkable similarities between placental tissue and cancer have led to the creation of a special centre dedicated exclusively to the study of the placenta—The Center for Trophoblast Research, at Cambridge University.

Another astonishing aspect of the placenta's behaviour is the fact that although it is an organ derived fifty percent from the father, it does not follow the usual transplant theory. Syncytiotrophoblast is a masked tissue: it is not recognized as an alien tissue by the mother. It is the only human tissue that lacks histocompatibility antigens, which identify a cell as being from one's self or not from one's self, determining whether a tissue graft will be accepted by an organ transplant recipient or not. In this way, the trophoblast can infiltrate and erode maternal vessels without being noticed. Thus, the mother's body is tricked into accepting what is actually an alien material (Loke).

PLACENTAL TRANSFUSION: THE IMPORTANCE OF WAITING

Why do we clamp and cut the umbilical cord before the birth of the placenta? (Hutchon). When did this practice begin to take place? Considering the fact that placentation in mammals occurred one hundred and forty million years ago, we can assume that nature has had enough time to perfect this process. So why do we think that this physiological event needs intervention? Is it for any practical reasons? Is it for easier management of the third stage of labour? Is it for pediatricians to examine the baby as soon as possible? Is it for legal worries? Is it the need to quickly check the cord blood in order to establish if there is anything wrong with the baby from delivery, thus discharging the gynaecologist from any responsibility? Is it for cultural reasons? Is there some fear of mother-infant bonding and, thus, of the primacy of the mother?

In our society, it seems that early maternal bonding is dreaded, or is seen as leading to dependency. It is as if early bonding to one's mother is regarded as a limitation for individual freedom, a bond to be quickly severed. Perhaps this is why some of the most significant biological steps that are naturally necessary to build bonds have become targets of obstetrical practices (Schmid).

This interest in the hypermanagement of umbilical cord clamping in Western culture began long ago, with Aristotle's publication of

Historia animalium in 369 BCE. In modern times, during the 1950s, the practice of early clamping became routine, as a consequence of the medicalization of birth. Two important trials by Bristol and Hinchingbrooke gave "definitive" conclusions to support this active management of the third stage of labour, which includes early clamping.[1] They demonstrated that this procedure reduced the incidence of postpartum haemorrhage (Prendville; Begley et al.).

Yet there is no scientific evidence that early clamping prevents postpartum blood loss. All recent literature states the contrary: delaying cord clamping reduces postpartum blood loss (Botha; Walsh; Fahy et al.; World Health Organization). When the umbilical cord is not clamped, the placenta can transfer its blood volume back to the baby (which is the baby's own blood), and, thus, the placenta will separate from the womb less traumatically. Today, we know that clamping the cord too early, within thirty seconds to one minute after the baby is born, deprives the newborn of about one third of her or his total blood volume, which is still circulating in the placenta. This is about one hundred and fifty millilitres of blood. This dramatic reduction of blood volume would have a severe outcome in any other moment of an individual's life (Morley). Newborns have an extraordinary capacity to adapt themselves, and in the majority of cases, no evident damage is done. Although it has no clear benefit and no rationale to support it, early cord clamping remains a too common practice among obstetricians and midwives in Western healthcare (Ononenze and Hutchon; Boere; Jelin et al.).

In addition, immediate cord clamping does not allow the baby to stabilize her or his cardiovascular system, because early clamping reduces the preload of blood to the heart by blocking forty percent of the venous return of blood from the placenta via the umbilical vein. At the same time, this increases the afterload of blood dramatically by obstructing the umbilical arteries, thus increasing peripheral vascular resistance (Van Vondereen et al., 2014). A recent study conducted on more than 150,000 newborns demonstrates how waiting to clamp the cord reduces about twenty percent of hospitalizations in paediatric pathology departments (Ersdal et al.). Why is this so? The fetus inside the womb is immersed in amniotic liquid. During the last weeks of pregnancy, the lungs produce half a litre of pulmonary liquid a day, a liquid that is similar to water. Pulmonary alveoli are surrounded by a capillary bed. During fetal life, alveoli are like collapsed spheres filled with pulmonary liquid. A new paradigm explaining neonatal transition physiology enlightens us about the importance of a complete placental transfusion: at birth, the capillary bed surrounding the alveoli is gradually perfused by blood coming from the placenta (Mercer and Skovgaard). Hydrostatic pressure expands the alveoli as a consequence of pressure rising because of the full expansion of the capillaries. In this way, the circulating blood drains the pulmonary liquid that occupies the lungs (Jaykka). Only after this drainage is complete can air fill the alveoli, allowing the baby to breath independently and gradually.

There is more. Late clamping provides the baby with forty to fifty percent additional red blood cells compared to early clamping, which means thirty-five to seventy-five milligrams of extra iron. A newborn needs 0.7 milligrams of iron per day for his growth and development. A complete placental transfusion provides enough iron for the first six months of life (Rabe et al.; Andersson et al.; Ceriani et al.). This time coincides with the most critical period of brain development, during which most the brain's neural pathways are established. Besides avoiding anemia, iron has long-term effects on the baby (Georgieff).

The only trial we know at present about the long-term effects of delayed cord clamping was published in 2015 by Andersson and others. This study proves that prevention of iron deficiency promotes neurodevelopment. Waiting three minutes before clamping the cord is associated with better fine motor skills and social skills in four-year-old children. Early clamping also deprives the baby of additional stem cells, which play an essential role in the development and maturity of many organ systems. Thus, the artificial loss of stem cells at birth could potentially affect later development and predispose infants to diseases, such as chronic lung disease, asthma, diabetes, epilepsy, cerebral palsy, Parkinson's disease, infection, and neoplasm. In particular, the postnatal transfer of umbilical cord blood cells may be important in preterm infants (Sanberg). The umbilical cord blood of infants born between twenty-four to thirty-one weeks gestation contains a higher concentration of primitive haematopoietic progenitor cells (Tolosa). This is why the practice of cord blood banking may be inappropriate. Immediate clamping (within thirty seconds) is the only way to make harvesting successful. At least fifteen billion nuclear cells have to be harvested to bank the blood . As such, why are we allowing the theft of all these important cells, the lifeblood of newborns? (Tolosa; Skoko; Díaz-Rossello).

PLACENTA, MATERNAGE, AND GENOMIC IMPRINTING: THE DIALOGUE BETWEEN BRAIN AND PLACENTA AND THE ROLE OF FATHERS

The amazing placenta has a fundamental and irreplaceable role in the reproductive success of the human species. Thanks to the existence of the placenta, the mother takes care of the offspring in her body and supports correct brain development. Thanks to her or his placenta, the offspring can suckle milk from the mother. The ability of the placenta to create a bond between mother and offspring is genetically programmed. The genes regulating this activity belong to a special gene's family: imprinted genes. Almost all of human imprinted genes are expressed in the placenta as well as in the central nervous system.

Genomic imprinting is an unusual mechanism of gene control known only in mammals and marsupials. This mechanism makes the two parental genomes different by silencing one of the two alleles (maternal or paternal) of some special genes: genes that have a regulatory function. In particular, they control placental and fetal growth. The existence of these genes is due to conflicting interests in mammals between the father and the mother. There is a marked parental difference in the assignment of resources intended for offspring growth. The placenta is the site for this mother-father genomic debate (Loke; Moore and Haig).

The father, and the imprinted genes paternally expressed, is interested in granting a big placenta for the fetus to access the maximum of food from the mother. The mother's interest, and the one of the imprinted genes maternally expressed, is to keep her resources for the sake of her own health and for her next pregnancies. This model explains why paternal imprinted genes promote placental growth whereas maternal imprinted genes limit such growth. It is in the balanced activation of paternal and maternal imprinted genes that a fine and physiological placentation occurs. The placenta should not grow too much or too little—a fine balance.

Another important aspect linked to genomic imprinting is a mechanism of crucial importance for the evolutionary success of "maternage." Recently, a special group of *imprinted genes* located on chromosome 19 have been studied in relation to maternal behaviour. This group of genes, called "Peg 3" (paternally expressed gene three), if mutated in mice, generates behavioural disorders in the mother (He and Joomyeong). She is not able to suckle the offspring, nor to thermo-regulate, nor to build her nest. Because of this, her offspring don't survive. The mammary glands are normal, but she is unable to eject milk. At the same time, offspring with mutant alleles are not able to suckle from their mothers—another astonishing discovery of how paternal contribution silently takes place, and may interfere with maternal biological functions (Keverne; Li et al.).

It is interesting to notice that the female fetus learns to respond to placenta imprinted genes during her stay into the mother's uterus. After a long period of latency, when she herself becomes pregnant as an adult, her answer to the imprinted genes will be more effective and rapid. Some studies have shown how even males, during their partner's pregnancies, undergo some important hormonal modifications stimulating how they care for the mother and the child. This behaviour may be a response to the effect, during males' fetal life, of the imprinted genes (Curley).

PLACENTOPHAGIA IN HUMANS AND MAMMALS: AN EVOLUTIONARY BEHAVIOUR

Why do mammals eat their placenta after delivery? Different hypotheses have been formulated to explain this particular behaviour. The most well-known reason is the need to clean the birth place, in order to avoid aggressive, blood-smelling predators. Another explanation is the need to quickly regain the life force after delivery, by eating this highly nutritional organ (Schwartz; Selander et al; Young and Benyshek).

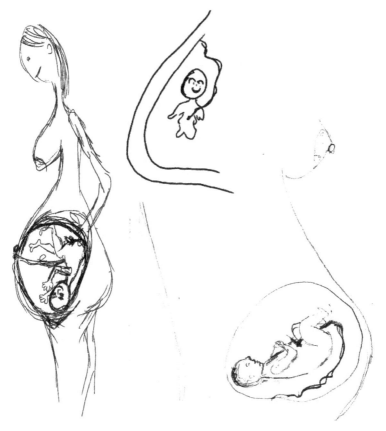

The missing placenta - pictures drawn by mothers.

Other studies have shown that mammals eat their placenta to prevent hemolytic disease of the newborn. Specifically, eating the placenta avoids the production of antibodies against fetal antigens, which represents an evolutionary advantage. Placentophagia is also immunologically beneficial, as ingestion of placenta may support immunization of the mother against the placental cells that remain in utero after birth and may, if not rejected, pose a threat to the mother's health (e.g., choriocarcinoma). Thus, eating placenta has other consequences. This organ contains a hormone called placental opioid-enhancing factor (POEFF), which enhances the opioid cerebral circuit of the mother. In other words, ingestion of placenta stimulates a feeling of wellbeing that helps the mother to quickly overcome fatigue after giving birth, and supports a loving and caring mood toward her offspring (Kristal).

THE VANISHING PLACENTA

I have tried to give a few scientific insights about the placenta—an intelligent and generous organ, capable of accomplishing so many different activities. This organ was venerated in many preindustrial cultures, so it is surprising how few people in Western cultures, particularly how few women, even pregnant ones, are aware of its importance. As a midwife, I have asked many expectant mothers to draw images for me of their womb, baby, and placenta. Some of their drawings are on page 137. Where has the amazing placenta gone? It is missing. I hope we can bring it back to modern consciousness, for the care and wellbeing of mothers and babies. And especially for the health of all human beings being born and coming into this amazing life.

ENDNOTES

[1]There is no general consensus about the timing of umbilical cord clamping. Several definitions can be found in scientific publications:
- •Immediate and early clamping: as soon as the newborn comes out of the birth canal to one minute
- •Late clamping: three minutes after birth to when the umbilical cord stops pulsating.
- •Mini lotus birth: clamping after placenta's delivery.
- •Lotus birth: no clamping; the umbilical cord falls off spontaneously several days after birth.

WORKS CITED

Andersson, Ola, et al., "Effect of Delayed versus Early Umbilical Cord Clamping on Neonatal Outcomes and Iron Status at 4 Months: A Randomised Controlled Trial." *British Medical Journal*, vol. 343, 2011.

Andersson, Ola, et al. "Effect of Delayed Cord Clamping on Neurodevelopment at 4 Years of Age, A Randomized Clinical Trial." *JAMA Pediatrics, vol.* 169, no. 7, 2015, pp. 631-638. The JAMA Network, doi: 10.1001/jamapediatrics.2015.0358.

Begley, CM, et al. "Active Versus Expectant Management for

Women in the Third Stage of Labour (Review)." *The Cochrane Database of Systematic Review*, no.3, 2015, pp. 1-157. *Cochrane Library*, doi: 10.1002/14651858.CD007412.pub4.

Boere, I., et al. "Current Practice of Cord Clamping in the Netherlands: A Questionnaire Study." *Neonatology*, vol. 107, no. 1, 2015, pp. 50-55.

Botha, M. C. "The Management of the Umbilical Cord in Labour." *South African Journal of Obstetrics and Gynecology*, August 1968, pp. 30-33.

Ceriani, Cernadas J.M., et al. "The Effect of Timing of Cord Clamping on Neonatal Venous Hematocrit Values and Clinical Outcome at Term: A Randomized, Controlled Trial." *Pediatrics*, vol. 117, no. 4, 2006, pp. 779-786.

Curley, J.P., et al. "Coadaptation in Mother and Infant Regulated by a Paternally Expressed Imprinted Gene." *Proceedings of the Royal Society of London*, vol. 271, no. 1545, 2004, pp. 1303-1309.

Díaz-Rossello, Jose Luis. "Early Umbilical Cord Clamping and Cord-Blood Banking." *The Lancet*, vol. 368, 2006, http://www.thelancet.com/pdfs/journals/lancet/PIIS0140-6736(06)69323-9.pdf. Accessed 22 Apr. 2017.

Ersdal, Hege L., et al. "Neonatal Outcome Following Cord Clamping After Onset of Spontaneous Respiration," *Pediatrics*, vol. 134, no. 2, 2014, pp. 265-272.

Fahy, K., et al. "Holistic Physiological Care Compared with Active Management of the Third Stage of Labour for Women at Low Risk of Postpartum Haemorrhage: a Cohort Study." *Women and Birth*, vol. 23, no. 4, 2010, pp.146-152.

Georgieff, Michael K. "Long-Term Brain and Behavioral Consequences of Early Iron Deficiency." *Nutrition Reviews*, vol. 69, no. 1, Nov 2011. *NCBI*, doi: 10.1111/j.1753-4887.2011.00432.x.

He, Hongzhi, and Kim Joomyeong. "Regulation and Function of the Peg3 Imprinted Domain." *Genomics Inform*, vol. 12, no. 3, 2014, pp. 105-113.

Hutchon, David. "Why Do Obstetricians and Midwives Still Rush to Clamp the Cord?" *British Medical Journal*, vol. 341, 2010. *BMJ*, doi: https://doi.org/10.1136/bmj.c5447.

Jaykka, S. "An Experimental Study of the Effect of Liquid Pressure Applied to the Capillary Network of Excised Fetal Lungs." *Acta Paediatrica*, vol. 46, no. 112, 1957, pp 1-91. *Wiley Online Library*, doi: 10.1111/j.1651-2227.1957.tb08648.x.

Jelin, Angie C., et al. "Obstetricians' Attitudes and Beliefs Regarding Umbilical Cord Clamping." *The Journal of Maternal-Fetal and Neonatal Medicine*, vol. 27, no.14, 2014, pp. 1457-1461.

Keverne, E. B. "Importance of the Matriline for Genomic Imprinting, Brain Development and Behaviour." *Philosophical Transactions of the Royal Society*, vol. 368, no. 1609, 2013. *NCBI*, doi: 10.1098/rstb.2011.0327.

Keverne, E. B. "Genomic Imprinting, Maternal Care, and Brain Evolution." *Hormones and Behaviour*, vol. 40, 2001, pp. 146-155.

Kristal, Mark B., et al. "Placentophagia in Humans and Nonhuman Mammals: Causes and Consequences." *Ecology of Food and Nutrition*, vol. 51, no. 3, 2012, pp. 177-197.

Kristal, Mark. B. "Placentophagia: A Biobehavioral Enigma." *Neuroscience and Biobehaviorial Reviews*, vol. 4, no. 2, 1980, pp. 141-150.

Li, L., et al. "Regulation of Maternal Behaviour and Offspring Growth by Paternally Expressed Peg." *Science*, vol. 284, no. 5412, 1999, pp. 330-334.

Loke, Y.W. *Life Vital's Link*. Oxford University Press, 2013.

Mercer, Judith S., and Rebecca L. Skovgaard. "Neonatal Transition Physiology: a New Paradigm." *Journal of Perinatal & Neonatal Nursing*, vol. 15, no. 4, 2002, pp. 56-75.

Moore, T., and D. Haig. "Genomic Imprinting in Mammalian Development: A Parental Tug-of-War." *Trends in Genetics*, vol. 7, 1991, pp. 45-49.

Morley, G.M. "Cord Closure: Can Hasty Clamping Injure the Newborn?" *OBG Management*, July 1998, pp. 29-36, http://www.whale.to/a/morley1.html. Accessed 22 Apr. 2017.

Ononenze, A.B., and David J. Hutchon. "Attitude of Obstetricians Towards Delayed Cord Clamping: A Questionnaire-based Study." *Journal of Obstetrical Gynaecology*, vol. 29, no. 3, 2009, pp. 223-224.

Rabe, H., et al. "Long-Term Follow-up of Placental Transfusion in Full-Term Infants." *JAMA Pediatrics*, vol. 169, no. 7, 2015, pp. 623-624.

Ryan, Frank. *Virolution*. Collins, 2009.

Sanberg et al., "Delayed Umbilical Cord Blood Clamping: First Line of Defense Against Neonatal and Age-Related Disorders" *Wulfenia*, vol. 26, no. 6, 2014, pp. 243-249.

Schmid, Verena. "I Canali Biologici e Genetici dell'Attaccamento Madre-Bambino." *D & D*, vol. 17, 1997, http://verenaschmid. eu/articoli/i-canali-biologici-e-genetici-dell-attaccamen-to-madre-bambino. 22 Apr. 2017.

Schwartz, S. "Maternal Placentophagy as an Alternative Medicinal Practice in the Postpartum Period." *Midwifery Today International Midwife*, vol. 110, 2014, pp. 28-29.

Selander, Jodi, et al. "Human Maternal Placentophagy: A Survey of Self-reported Motivations and Experiences Associated with Placenta Consumption." *Ecology of Food and Nutrition*, vol. 52, no. 2, 2013, pp. 93-115.

Skoko, Elena. "Aspetti Pratici, Economici ed etici della Raccolta del Sangue Neonatale." *Academia.edu*, 2016, http://www.academia. edu/13450968/Aspetti_pratici_economici_ed_etici_della_rac-colta_del_sangue_neonatale. Accessed 22 Apr. 2017.

Tolosa, Jose N., et al. "Mankind's First Natural Stem Cell Transplant." *Journal of Cellular and Molecular Medicine*, vol. 14, no. 3, 2010, pp 488-495.

Van Vonderen J., et al., "Measuring Physiological Changes During the Transition to Life After Birth," *Neonatology*, vol.105 no. 3, 2014, pp. 230-242.

World Health Organisation. *Guideline: Delayed Umbilical Cord Clamping for Improved Maternal and Infant Health and Nutrition*. WHO, 2014.

World Health Organisation. *Recommendations for the Prevention and Treatment of Postpartum Haemorrhage: Evidence Base*. WHO 2012.

Young, Sharon M., and Daniel C. Benyshek. "In Search of Human Placentophagy: A Cross Cultural Survey of Human Placenta Consumption, Disposal Practices, and Cultural Beliefs." *Ecology of Food and Nutrition*, vol. 49, no. 6, 2010, pp. 467-484.

12.
Placental Thinking

The Gift of Maternal Roots

NANÉ JORDAN

I did not set out to learn about placentas. The afterbirth was an afterthought in my birth and mothering experience, grassroots work, and theory making. I became an avid and early student of what was the lay midwifery movement in Canada (Shroff), after attending the homebirth of my little brother in 1980s Toronto. I worked as a homebirth midwife's assistant, a hospital birth doula, and a postpartum home caregiver. We used the word "lay" to denote midwives in Canada and the United States who practised through community-based efforts and grassroots activism, from at least the 1970s onwards. Without legal status, women trained themselves in the art and science of midwifery through various means, including studying obstetrical textbooks, working with supportive doctors, travelling to birth clinics in other countries, doing apprenticeships with experienced midwives, and learning from birth itself. Through attending mothers giving birth at home, this movement restored natural, physiologic, low-tech birth giving to mothers and families.

My aims are multiple but interconnected in this chapter. I move from birth practice to maternal social theory and activism as I speak to the power of midwifery and woman-centred and mother-centred birth. I describe placenta structure and function, and share placenta practices from my early birth-study days. Finally, I play with ideas for what I am calling "placental thinking," as related to the maternal gift economy as theorized by philosopher Genevieve Vaughan. I explore the birth-*gifting* relations of mother-centred birth care, which is (by nature) at the heart of placental thinking.

I suggest that mother-centred care is always possible, no matter the place and manner of birth gifting.

As a woman-centred philosophy of care, midwifery holds mothers and babies at the centre of birth, which supports women's power, rights, choices and self-sufficiency, through honouring and loving women and babies. Pregnancy and birth are understood to be normal lifecycle events. Support from an experienced midwife can help mothers to holistically navigate the experiences of pregnancy, birth, and postpartum and to maintain optimal health and wellbeing not only in the physical dimensions of birth but in the mental, emotional, and spiritual ones as well. "Holistic," thus, refers to the whole person as a multifaceted being. With available medical backup as needed, midwifery care is possible for most healthy women. I became an early promoter of home and natural childbirth, and the amazing physiology that is inherent in birth. I witnessed over and over the courage of mothers, and the self-empowering, healing, and even ecstatic spiritual potentials of giving birth (Buckley; Young).

In particular, North American mothers and midwives were discovering and recovering from the intervention-focused, paternalistic, and hierarchical limitations of the medical system in regards to holistic and woman-centred care (Arms). One limitation—only fully realized after others, such as episiotomy, lithotomy position, and strapping of limbs—was the lack of connection between birthing mothers and their babies' placentas. Umbilical cords were and still are cut quickly, and once born, placentas were and are immediately removed from mother and baby to be disposed of. Mothers may not be fully aware of this organ, which has been an integral part of the growth of their own baby. Or there may be an aversion to or disinterest in its mysterious, blood-filled mass. It is true that the bloody placenta is the only organ that willingly exits a human body once its life-giving purpose is fulfilled, still attached to the human it sustained. Yet the placenta as a real, physical and meaningful aspect of pregnancy and birth was and is undervalued. This was and is not well understood in mainstream medical economies of birth.

The most common treatment of the placenta is as blood waste or as medical property for research purposes. For many mothers, the placenta may appear as the final byproduct of birth—as refuse or something left for others to use or dispose of at an institutional level. As theorized by anthropologist Robbie David-Floyd, this kind of birth practice is a form of ritual. Ritual can be any continuous action or sociocultural practice that establishes key orders and regulations of thought, materials, or services. In this case, the medical ritual disconnects mothers and babies postbirth from each other and their placentas. Mothers and midwives, in what was the midwifery and homebirth movement, were vicariously rediscovering and learning about babies' placentas. They were also discovering birth-giving powers and strengths that had been disparaged or hidden, much like the humble placenta itself.

RELATIONAL DESIGNS

As a young midwives' assistant, I became used to cleaning up and disposing of the blood naturally shed in birth. I was also learning how to handle and care for placentas during and after birth. I knew that the placenta had to be born in a timely way, that the umbilical cord was not cut until it had stopped pulsing, and that the placenta must appear whole without missing pieces. I especially remember the first time I was taught how to "read" a placenta up close. Learning with an experienced midwife, I peered curiously at the bright red placenta she brought from a recent birth in all its blood-red glory. Through close instruction, I began to see, to discern its shape. I was soon in awe of this seemingly sacred design and structure.

There are two sides to a placenta: a mother side and a baby side. The mother side has groups of intersecting lobes that appear almost brainlike. The mother side attaches to the inside wall of her uterine muscle, connecting her life blood toward her baby's nourishment. The baby side is full of roots, roots, roots—in networks of veins and arteries. They interconnect lacelike, fanning outwards in a circular pattern from the umbilical cord, which attaches itself near the centre of the placental mass. The baby side is smooth and cosseted by the amniotic sack, which rises from the edges of the placenta to surround the baby in utero. During pregnancy, the placenta is the key developmental link between mother and child. The umbilical cord transports blood from baby toward and away from the mother through the vascular root system of the placenta. Via placental interchange through capillary diffusion, nourishment and oxygen are drawn from the body of the mother while metabolic wastes are released from the baby for the mother to dispose of. The placenta is singular in its mission: it grows and is born to support and sustain the life of the new human in and from the body of the mother.

It was not until after years of attending homebirths, working intimately with mothers and babies postbirth, and handling many placentas that I began to glean the morphological and spiritual wonders of this generative organ. Like a grand communicator, the placenta and umbilical cord define the paradox of the two bodies' connection and separation. The placenta grows like an apparatus from the baby itself, facilitating a continual dialogue of blood with the mother. Our first language is truly one of maternal nourishment, which flows from mother to child in a heart-to-heart rhythm—an abundant mother stream that ensures the baby's growth and survival. As a relational interface, this is not a fusion of bodies but a unilateral "gift" communication from mother to baby.

Because of my studies and graduate research in women's spirituality, I began to name the importance of the birth knowledge and wisdom that I had been privy to. I committed to writing and research that could transmit what I and others knew about birth, seeking to expand understandings of social philosophy from birth-based perspectives, which were missing from the Western philosophical tradition—dominated as this is by male-centered thinking that does not take birth experience into account. In this tradition, birth and birth giving are devalued and accorded lower value than social, cultural, and spiritual production, as if mothers and birth are not connected to social and cultural life at its core (O'Brien). Birth mysteries have been invariably silenced, lost, or co-opted through socialized and patriarchal disconnections of our birth-based origins from actual mothers and women. As a foundational experience of human life, revisioning birth in mother-centred ways can provide socially transformative values. In this, I aim for a society that supports, values, and loves mothers, babies, and children at the centre of life rather than at the social and economic peripheries. I aim for this not to essentialize women only as birth givers but to liberate mothers toward the meaning and leadership that is theirs at the core of life.

PLACENTAL PRACTICES

Attending to placentas and cords during and after birth was an outgrowth of the kinds of holistic midwifery care and grassroots homebirth practices that I learned from. Midwives and mothers were following body wisdom in allowing birth to unfold—reclaiming what I would now call "mother- or matricentric" healing traditions. During my experiences learning with midwives, we used to think and read about issues relating to how women's knowledge had been lost or suppressed in Western societies over the ages—this included feminist readings about the historical impact of the European witch hunts on women's social practices and wisdom (Spretnak) and about the violent colonial impact on Indigenous cultures (Shiva). Through the collective midwifery movement, a large amount of study, intuition, trust, love, and decolonizing attunement continues to be at work.

So much of what we learned in those early midwifery years is flowing and flowering into mother- and baby-centred practices and uses of placentas—including not clamping or cutting the umbilical cord too soon and allowing it to stop pulsing, so all of the baby's blood can transfuse from the placenta back into baby itself. When the cord is left on its own, the natural physiology of birth, developed over millennia, completes itself. Not cutting the umbilical also means keeping mother and baby together, where they can touch, smell, see, hear, and meet each other—the hormonal physiology of bonding is at work.

Homebirth mothers often chose to bury their placentas. This might be done under a tree, in a yard, or in a park, somewhere close to where the baby was born. Families and midwives have created rituals and ceremonies with the placenta, giving thanks for the gift of life in the new baby, and thanks to the Earth. The other use, which still shocks many people, is to prepare, cook, and feed the mother some placenta postbirth, just as many mammals do. Placentas are hormone and nutrient rich; they balance and mediate mothers' physical and emotional wellbeing postbirth

146

(Enning). During my midwifery studies, we taught ourselves the technique of drying the placenta to make capsules of its powder, before this was known as "placental encapsulation," a practice that is now taking off across North America (Selander). Placenta capsules are understood to restore vitality and strength, and to support postpartum depression and/or have general therapeutic value during the long challenges of early mothering and beyond. Researchers have been investigating the regenerative properties of stem cells from placental blood for curing various diseases, making placentas a material of healing interest for medicine beyond the birth room (Parolini).

Attending homebirths, I also began a practice of keeping a piece of the baby's cord for mothers postbirth, as I would dry these in spiral shapes. The cord takes days or even weeks to dry out, and shrinks down in size. The umbilical cord is the original thread that ties us to the beginnings of life, an energetic metaphor that goes on long afterward. I have my own daughters' cords and umbilical stumps, dried in this fashion, and have kept them in special pouches. I also learned of homebirth mothers who practised "lotus birth," which means not cutting the cord at all. Lotus birth mothers keep the placenta with the baby intact for several days until the cord naturally dries up and falls away on its own. One must carefully wash, wrap, and care for the placenta in this case. It is thought to be physically and energetically gentle for the baby to keep the placenta until the cord releases itself (Lim).

Another artful, creative practice has been the "placenta print," which involves taking the afterbirth and some white paper, and directly printing the blood outlines of its mass onto the page. One makes a placenta print of each side, mother and baby. I love birth art for its many growing and evolving forms as creative expressions for mothers' experiences and honouring of birth and life (Lin).

PLACENTAL THINKING IN THE GIFT

My favourite placental metaphor is the tree. While raising my children on the West Coast of Canada, immersed in the coastal rainforests of our home, we have frequently observed gigantic overturned trees, blown over after big storms. These have incredibly splayed root systems, which get exposed when upturned, often reaching a whole story over our heads. Huge tree roots spread through circular clods of earth. From my midwifery studies, I recognized this familiar structure—a placental structure—on a massive scale. Like the veins and arteries of the placenta, tree roots filter into soil, seeking and exchanging nutrients, water, and succor from the Earth as Mother. This is just as we reached for nourishment from the bodies of our mothers, through latticelike roots of the placenta. In this amazing organic symmetry, our bodies incarnate a treelike form. I love to mediate upon and return to this image of the tree (of life) to understand the ecology of our lives and our interconnected origins with other beings. I see this as an embodied poetics that expresses gratitude and relationship to the trees, the earth, and the gift of life itself—an experience of Indigenous philosophy in the expressive notation of "all my relations."

From this vein or root of thought, I have been developing an application of what I would call "placental thinking," with a nod toward Sara Ruddick's *Maternal Thinking*. Maternal thinking recognizes the compelling intellectual work of mothering and its practice. It dispels the notion that motherhood is biologically determined or a purely instinctual occupation. Placental thinking understands placentas as being of great value and note, and extends the metaphor of placentas into mother-centred social philosophies and understandings.

An application for placental thinking grows from my reading of the maternal gift economy work of feminist, matricentric (mother-centred) philosopher Genevieve Vaughan. Vaughan's work on mothering as a gift economy realizes that the gifting work that mothers do provides the "free" infrastructure for our entire social fabric. The gift is understood to be a one-way process, where materials and services flow from mother to child. Gifts are given, freely, as the giver does not expect rewards. In this way, mothers provide what children require for growth and wellbeing. This is unlike the exchange economy, which requires payment or reward from the receiver for any services or goods rendered. By difference, in the gift economy, the receiver is accorded the value by virtue of being given the gifts. Gifts are not exchanged but given through taking turns in giving gifts. Vaughan expands upon her theory in

The Gift in The Heart of Language. She outlines the ways in which early language acquisition is rooted in this maternal gift economy. Babies develop communication through mirroring their mothers in practices of taking turns in giving gifts.

Strikingly, mothers' gift giving is first accomplished by the placenta in utero. The placenta embodies what I would call a "gift morphology"—with its rootlike vascular system that draws nourishment from the mother into the developing fetus in a one-way gifting of life blood. The mother's body cleans up waste products and toxins from her baby via the placenta. This job is continued postbirth as the mother feeds baby via breast or bottled milk, and monitors the baby's urination and bowel movements.

The breast itself is an almost external placenta. Each breast has a treelike structure where vascular networks are held in soft tissues that produce nutritious milk from the body of the mother. The communication for milk production is physiologically cued by the baby and the mother's response to baby. The timing and length of feeding activates the amount of milk that is produced by the mother. Through this flow of nourishment to baby, the mother provides yet another gift morphology. This relationship now includes a new flow and flowering of language through verbal, nonverbal, and body-centred communication between mother and baby. Especially poignant are expressions of affection through touching, holding, smiling, hugging, and kissing from mother to baby, and vice versa. Babies express their needs by tone of voice and physical actions, cueing specificities of care from their mothers. Children become more and more themselves through mirroring and response, self-expression, and mothers' attentions and interactions with them. Communication is central to building the fabric of a new person's social life, based from these early gifting relations.

This early maternal gift economy does not approximate the exchange economy, where something is only given in exchange for something else. A child requires the mother's immediate and constant giving, or the child will perish. The gift is also present in the Earth's resources as a continual free stream of goods that humans need. Yet much of human life is being commodified through exchange and market economies. Work, services, and the "free" goods of the Earth itself have costs in their exchange value. Greed is common in the market economy, especially as corporations attempt to own everything, which renders invisible the original gifts—the trees, the earth, or the mothers.

I follow Vaughan's understanding of how gift and exchange economies are interlinked systems. The market economy needs the free gifts and resources of the gift economy. Mothers produce communicative bodies that eventually become the labour force for the market economy. We grow up inside the gift economies of our maternal and family relations, and whatever levels of gifting or exchange interactions and amassing of goods and services our families and societies provide us. For example, in societies such as Canada, the common people and governments currently value primary education and healthcare as being mostly "free" for all. This does not mean that these services do not cost anything, but they are made available as gifts to all to strengthen the wellbeing of the whole population. In other societies, such services are in the hands of forces of exchange, and may become subject to profit driven schemes rather than being seen as a social good or gift. In general, societies with higher gift-centred economies and, thus, mother-centred and placental-thinking economies, enjoy a stronger social fabric. When taken to its fullest, the gifting placental economy could function very well on its own, without the market. At its core, gifting is the foundation of life and love in action. However, the market cannot survive without the gifts of life, instead too often becoming a parasite on the gift—enslaving others to enforce gifts as extractions of resources at the cost of life and love. At its core, gifting is the foundation of life and love in action.

BIRTH GIFTING: MOTHERS AT THE CENTRE

Through placental relations and placental thinking, we can imagine this gift economy as located in the heart of the primal mother-baby dyad. There, I would locate a specific embodied maternal order of the gift that flows from mother to child, and onward into the whole social milieu, as life goes on from this primal, primary relationship. As Genevieve Vaughan notes, there are many hidden ways of the gift that are not yet named. I thus name the placenta, with its gift morphology (growth, structure, and design), as an embodied gift economy that has always existed. The eventual maternal act and power of giving birth flow from placental relations. Beyond the birth process, mother and child are released from their in-utero placental bonds and set off on the trajectory of new mother-child gifting relations.

In the current market system and exchange economy, placentas are literally thrown out after birth. This is a striking action and metaphor for our social understandings of the maternal gift as being literally worthless. The notion of garbage itself is "refuse" or what is refused. Thus, the gift is refused and made invisible. Mothers know little about their babies' placentas, often never seeing them in the hospital except for as a bloody lump in a metal side tray left aside after the birth. In the exchange economy, value is only apparent when the market assigns value to the placenta, as in its use for stem cell research or in the cosmetics industry. We could read this in newspapers and hardly connect stem cells to the placentas of our own early lives, born from our mothers' bodies and blood. The association of birth blood with refuse also relates to long-time taboos, secrecy, and shame associated with menstrual blood in Western cultures (Grahn). Rather than socially upholding the sacred function of the female body's life-gifting powers, the public prefers the death blood dominate in popular media culture, and the lived realities of violence and war. In contrast, the blood of life and birth receives silent attention.

Further separation rituals, such as early cord cutting and taking the baby away from the mother at the moment of birth, disrupt mother-baby bonding, hormonal systems, and unity. These procedures ultimately interrupt the physiological peak of mothers' experiences of relief, pleasure, and love in birth gifting, which are part of early bonding and begin the moment a mother becomes pregnant (Buckley). There is an intended dynamic of "safe" birth care at work in obstetrical practices in order to diminish the risks of birth giving. Ostensibly, doctors work in concert with medical protocols and interventions to ward off the risk and fear of death and feelings of pain—truisms of birth. Mothers and babies do walk along the edges of life and death in birth's passage, in which giving birth is an overwhelming experience that can be painful or dangerous, and requires our whole sense of being. The life-saving capacities of modern medicine are important in this regard. Yet it appears that through fear of pain and death, dominant authoritative structures have become linked to the medicalization of birth and the overuse of interventions. Fear of entering an overwhelming experience such as birth, and often without support, education, understanding, or some attending human warmth and kindness, may also be keeping people tied to a system that loses sight of the maternal gift. Also lost are the positive experiential potentials for relief and even pleasure in giving birth through one's own power and agency. As we continue to apply medical technologies and market-based, hierarchical attitudes of authority in birth care, can we shift birth practices toward more giftlike ways? Can we put mothers and babies at the centre of birth gifting through placental thinking?

In midwifery, a "motherer,"as Genevieve Vaughan names it, is anyone who satisfies needs unilaterally, not expecting reward. Is this a missing or lost gift economy in birth? Of course, there are doctors who practice this gift, putting mothers and babies at the centre of birth, who view mothers kindly and lovingly with care. But directing the gift of compassionate attention is a more common philosophy for midwives and doulas, which includes the ability and commitment to support and empathize with the mother. In a diagrammatic perspective, this looks like a circle, with supportive caregivers holding space for the mother, who is at the centre. In this circle, the mother can retain and direct her own energies and agency for birth giving, both physical and psychic, toward herself and her baby. She is in trusting relations with her attendants, who direct their energy toward her (and not themselves) as needed, and have ability to step back if not needed. In authoritarian and hierarchical systems of care, the energy of birth is directed in straight lines up and away from the mother and baby and toward the attendants at the top. Attention tends to focus on the birth attendants as they dictate the directions for birth experience and implement their expertise, often without regard for the mothers' wishes. Mothers may feel depleted or worse, traumatized from giving birth under systems that appropriate their birth-gifting power without regard for the centrality of their agency and experience. Obviously, there are many nuances and complexities to this topic, and often more analysis is needed on a case-by-case basis.

In this regard, birth giving inherently asks a mystery of us. It is older and wiser than our clocks and interventions, and unfolds uniquely for every mother and baby who enter its experience. I have witnessed home and hospital births with "motherer" attendants at hand, where those mothers and babies are held at the centre of a circle of care and love. Attendants keep a respectful watch, moving toward or away as asked or needed. A birthing mother, feeling safe to surrender into her own birth process—however this is for her as she navigates pain, body sensation, pleasure, mind and emotion of it all—exudes her own hormonal cocktail. Birthing energies, generated by mother and baby, can instill a sense of grace in the birth room as baby arrives, earth side.

Thus, placental thinking is enacted in holistic and empowering models of woman-centred birth, which value mothers' integrity and wellbeing. At home, in clinics, birth centres or hospitals, anywhere really, mother- and baby- centred care is always advisable and possible, no matter the interventions or procedures that are needed (World Health Organization). This gifting of care through a socially just attitude depends heavily on the people, philosophies, and practices in these places. Placental thinking moves beyond patriarchal, authoritarian, market-based practices of birth toward valuation of mothers and the experiential gifts and gifting of life.

CONCLUDING PLACENTAL GIFTS

Reclaiming the role and value of the placenta may help transform our understandings of birth and return human origins to the mother. Becoming a placental thinker, I call for new science, arts, and understandings of birth to arise from social movements of birth, from mothers' direct birthing experiences, and from the wisdom that is deeply embedded in mothers, birth givers, and humans being born. We would not be here without the eons of human birthing relationships that have come before us, nor without the stream of mother gifts that predates our own lives. We are given the gift, and we can pass this gift to others. The passing along of gifts is most poignant in the opposite of birth—death. Placental thinking speaks to the fundamental necessity of human regeneration. We are durational beings that die and require the next generation to be given life to go on.

I honour the sacred gift of life that comes from so many birthings, which includes attention to our human interrelationship with the Earth as Mother, from which we draw continually and return all the gifts of our life force and source. In such ways, the placenta is making its wisdom known among mothers and others. Worldwide, mother-gifting pathways can be traced, claimed, and followed for the sustenance and affirmation of life, which is at the maternal roots of our human being and doing.

WORKS CITED

Arms, Suzanne. *Immaculate Deception II: Myth, Magic, and Birth*. Celestial Arts, 1996.
Buckley, Sarah. *Gentle Birth, Gentle Mothering*. One Moon Press, 2005.
Davis-Floyd, Robbie. *Birth as an American Rite of Passage*. University of California Press, 1992.
Enning, Cornelia. *Placenta: Gift of Life. The Role of the Placenta in Different Cultures and How to Prepare and Use it as Medicine*. Motherbaby Press, 2007.
Grahn, Judy. *Blood, Bread, and Roses: How Menstruation Created the World*. Beacon Press, 1993.
Lim, Robin. *Placenta: the Forgotten Chakra*. Half Angel Press, 2010.
Lin, Wennifer. *Birth Art and the Art of Birthing: Creation and Procreation on the Äina of Tütü Pele*. Dissertation, University of California, 2008.
O'Brien, Mary. *The Politics of Reproduction*. Routledge, 1981.
Parolini, Ornella, editor. *Placenta: The Tree of Life / Gene and Cell Therapy*. CRC Press /Productivity Press, 2016.
Ruddick, Sara. *Maternal Thinking: Towards a Politics of Peace*. Beacon Press, 1989.
Selander, Jodi. "Placenta Benefits Info: Avoid the Baby Blues." *Placenta Benefits*, http://placentabenefits.info. Accessed 10 Oct. 2016.
Shiva, Vandana. "Development as a Project of Western Patriarchy."

Reweaving the World: The Emergence of Ecofeminism, edited by Irene Diamond and Gloria Feman Orenstein, Sierra Club Books, 1990, pp.189-200.

Shroff, Farah. *The New Midwifery: Reflections on Renaissance and Regulation.* Women's Press, 1997.

Spretnak, Charlene, editor. *The Politics of Women's Spirituality: Essays on the Rise of Spiritual Power within the Feminist Movement.* Anchor Press/Doubleday, 1982.

Vaughan, Genevieve, editor. *Il dono/The gift.* Meltemi editore, 2004.

Vaughan, Genevieve. *The Gift in the Heart of Language: The Maternal Source of Meaning.* Mimesis International, 2015.

Vaughan, Genevieve, editor. *Women and the Gift Economy: A Radically Different Worldview is Possible.* Inanna Publications, 2007.

World Health Organization (WHO). "Human Reproduction Program. Sexual and Reproductive Health—Prevention and Elimination of Disrespect and Abuse in Childbirth" WHO, http://www.who.int/reproductivehealth/topics/maternal_perinatal/statement-childbirth-govnts-support/en/. Accessed 22 Nov. 2016.

Young, Cathrine, editor. *Mother's Best Secrets.* Mother Press, 1992.

Artful Pause II

ARTWORK BY
AMANDA GREAVETTE AND NANÉ JORDAN

The Birth Project

AMANDA GREAVETTE

THE BIRTH PROJECT by Amanda Greavette is a series of paintings depicting women, birth, and motherhood. These life-size paintings represent the real and symbolic nature of birth as a holistic experience. Birth is a powerful and profound event that changes and shapes one's identity. The physical, emotional, and spiritual awakening of giving birth is the perfect landscape to explore universal experiences like pain, euphoria, transformation, and the welcoming of new life. The artist aims to create work that is provocative, beautiful, and heavy with emotion and symbol. Although Amanda paints birth because she loves it, she wants the paintings and their images to creatively and effectively tell women's stories as experienced in everyday life.

As a body of artwork, the Birth Project is intended to inspire confidence and possibility in women who are approaching pregnancy and motherhood by portraying these experiences in real and tangible ways. These paintings fill a visual void in birth culture by promoting positive and empowering images of childbirth and motherhood. The artist wishes to raise public awareness of issues surrounding birth and to contribute to a social dialogue and movement that creates positive changes for childbearing women. The Birth Project has been exhibited at galleries and conferences around North America. It is a continually changing exhibition as the series develops with new artwork. Submissions are accepted on an ongoing basis for those who'd like to participate with their photos and stories. To find out more about the Birth Project, please visit: www.amandagreavette.com; http://amandagreavette.blogspot.com. Or find the "Amanda Greavette Fine Art" community on Facebook and Etsy.

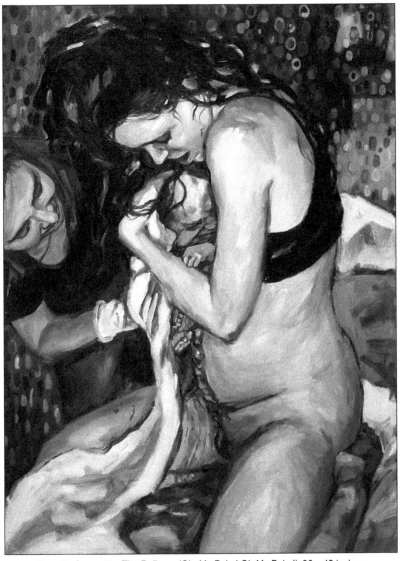

Amanda Greavette, *The Delivery (Oh, My Baby! Oh My Baby!)*, 36 x 48 inches, oil on canvas, 2008-2010

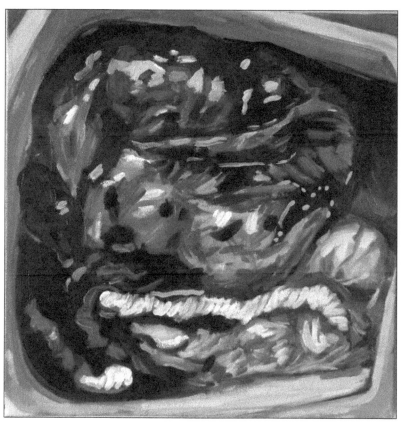

Amanda Greavette, *Placenta—Tree of Life*, 12 x 12 inches, oil on canvas, 2011

The Placenta Project

NANÉ JORDAN

I SOUGHT AN AESTHETIC DREAMING RESPONSE for what I was
discovering in communication about, and communion with, birth
and placentas. In my textile artwork, I spin, dye, and weave with
red thread to express my affinity for women's blood power and
agency through our experiences of pregnancy, birth giving, and
mothering. I wanted to visually translate the life-giving intensity
of this blood colour and substance that I had witnessed over and
over through attending births as a midwifery apprentice. I, thus,
created a series of life-size placental forms by dying wool with
various hues of rich-red colours. To make these forms, I used a
wool-felting technique to create a series of felted placentas with
long homespun wool for umbilical cords.

Upon creating a dozen felted placental forms with trailing umbilici, I began installing them in the environs of the Toronto Islands
in Lake Ontario, just offshore from the city of Toronto—my own
birthplace. Thus was born, *The Placenta Project*, as I connected
placental forms to trees and water in natural settings, and umbilical cords that reached down to the earth as "Mother." My
placenta placements emerged as dots or *bindis*, marking trees and
water as sacred sites. Depending on my placements, they became
choruses of branching, umbilical-gestating activity, or they floated
serenely in the womblike water of the lake, dwelling as if from
watery origins. As a birth-based artistic inquiry, *The Placenta
Project* births relational events of interconnection among elements
of trees, vegetation, sandy shorelines, and water. I am reflecting
upon the centrality of gestation, growth, and birth in human and

natural life, which includes my desire to express reciprocity with all mothers and the Earth as Mother, through placental relations.

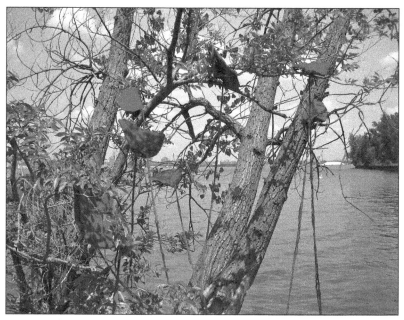

Nané Jordan, *The Placenta Project 1*, textile placements & photography, 2010

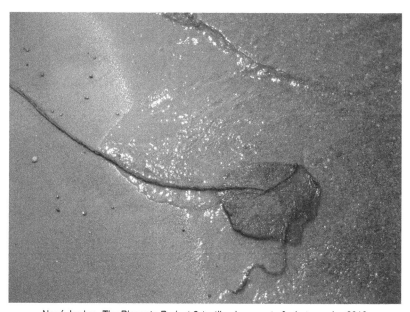

Nané Jordan, *The Placenta Project 2*, textile placements & photography, 2010

PLACENTERRE III

13.
Bledsung of the Placenta

Women's Blood Power
at the Sacred Roots of Economics

POLLY WOOD

Menstruation is blood's secret name. All blood is menstrual blood.—Judy Grahn (*Blood, Bread, and Roses* viii)

WHAT DO PLACENTAS HAVE IN COMMON with economics? How can understanding the relationship between the two shed light on the importance of the power in women's bloodshed? If we look at placentas from the role that women's blood rituals play in the global economy, will we see the value of creating a relationship to placentas that treats them in a sacred way?

Based on my research of economic theory, as well as metaformic theory, I have learned that the roots of economics were not about money but about the shedding of blood and how we cared for and managed what was "sacred" to us. Metaformic theory proposes a cross-cultural origin story of human consciousness that restores menstrual rituals to the centre of culture. In this way, awakening to consciousness was held sacred. Carefully and ritually keeping the order of things was a way to *remind* ourselves of beginnings, lest we fall back into chaos. Metaformic theory's famed cultural theorist, Judy Grahn, posits that our ancient bleeding sisters followed menstrual seclusion rites in order to reenact the original awakening of human consciousness (*Blood, Bread* 17). Grahn writes the following: "Origin stories remember a time before anything was, a time that consisted entirely of darkness, of water, of endless space, or of flatness without landscape; a time before name, before consciousness; a time described as asleep, or dreaming, or by the Greek word *chaos*, meaning 'yawning'" (7).

Before humans measured the monetary value of things, we measured time. Counting time was practised before counting shells, grain, coins, or dollars. Our earliest ancestors etched lines in bone and stone. They counted time by marking the light and dark cycles of the moon as well as their cycles of menstruation and birth, which were synchronized to the lunar cycles. "Currency" is a word commonly use in economics describing an agreed-upon measurement for a specific kind of money or medium of exchange, but the roots of the word are synonymous with bloodshed: "The etymon of 'currency' is from the Latin *currentum* 'condition of flowing,' and of *currere* 'to run'" (Wood 42).

I imagine what it may have been like to be one of our earliest prehuman ancestors living on the edge of awakening between chaos and consciousness. I imagine learning to value the carefully managed rituals of those around me, whose blood came freely flowing, right when the gradually decreasing light of the moon left nothing but darkness. I imagine that after a time of bleeding in the dark, I notice them emerging from seclusion, just as the light of the moon appears. If conception had occurred prior to the dark of the moon, a new level of awakening was born as well. For along with the halting of this consciousness-bringing bloodshed, a belly slowly swelled like the moon itself, and there was something new to measure. While new life grew alongside the placenta within, I imagine being curious of whether or not one had actually swallowed the light of the moon. I wonder, after enough cycles of light and darkness had passed and the new life was born, just how that sacred, bloody placenta would be cared for and managed.

PLACENTA POWER

I have been working hands on with placentas for six years now. When I began birth work as a doula in the late 1990s, I simply thought of the placenta as something poetic and as the soul twin of the new baby. Once after assisting a birth, I was asked to make prints of the tree-of-life image, which appears on the fetal side of the placenta. It seemed like a natural extension of the visual birth art I was creating in my free time. I knew about the placenta's ability to feed the baby and carry away waste as its main function, but it was not until many years later that I began to understand just how amazing this organ really is and how the way in which placentas are cared for speaks volumes about how our global economic system values women's blood rituals.

My current work with placentas would not be possible without the inspiration that came during a 2009 trip to Toronto to attend a conference called "A (M)otherworld is Possible: Two Feminist Visions." I had stepped away from assisting at births after the birth of my own daughter in 2002, and before she had turned a year old, I returned to college to complete my undergraduate work, of which I had begun ten years prior. It was during that academic return, at the California Institute of Integral Studies in San Francisco, that I began writing about the value of my experience in birth work. As I continued on to graduate school at New College of California in 2004, I created music as well as literary, visual, and performance art based on women's cross-cultural rites of passage and, more specifically, on women's blood rituals.

During the (M)otherworld conference in Toronto, which was a gathering of feminist motherhood scholars, the matriarchal studies global community, as well as the International Feminists for the Study of the Gift Economy, I was reintroduced to the power of placentas through a beautiful presentation by Nané Jordan called, "A Poetics of the Placenta: Placental Cosmology as Gift and Sacred Economy." In a published version of the paper, Jordan writes that "Every time a mother or family reclaims their placenta, acknowledges through ceremony, preparations, and women's medicine practices, its role in gifting the 'life' of their child, a larger connection to the cosmos, to the earth community is made" (282). This was a pivotal moment for me, both in my history of birth work as well as in my developing contributions to the understanding of the "blood economy." Nané's presentation helped me find my way back into the embodied birth work that I deeply love and into the new branch of it that I currently offer.

As a professional Placenta Encapsulation Specialist, I serve women in the first weeks after giving birth through the postpartum support process of encapsulating the placenta for ingestion, a technique based on traditional Chinese medicine. This modern, standardized process, which was pioneered by the research and training organization Placenta Benefits, increases a woman's wellness after the birth of her baby by giving her energy and an emotional buoyancy; increasing her milk supply; helping her uterus contract; reducing anxiety; and, generally, contributing to her overall sense of nourishment (Selander).

Being with new mothers in the first few days postpartum and keeping closely in touch in the weeks following gives me an opportunity to share useful resources and offer additional support in the mental and emotional realm. The shift in focus from the pregnant and birthing mother to the new baby can often leave the mother depleted during an extremely selfless and self-giving time. The nourishment and care of mothers during what is considered the often-invisible "fourth trimester" is essential to their overall health and ability to take care of their babies.

I would not be doing this amazing work if it were not for the inspiration I received at the (M)otherworld conference during Nané's presentation. I was moved to tears while listening and watching, all the while remembering my passionate connection to hands-on birth work. This was the work I had stepped away from to make room for my own birth as well as my move, eventually, into the academic realm and into a place of writing, dancing, and singing about birth and women's blood rites. "A Poetics of the Placenta" reignited my desire to be involved in birth work in a practical and embodied way. Now I serve women and their families during the childbearing years while carrying with me an understanding of the value of placentas in the larger context of women's cross-cultural rites of passage and blood rituals.

BLOOD ART ACTIVISM

I had been invited to be a conference performer at that gathering in Toronto, and offered some of my songs, presenting them in a style of "edu-tainment" that is enveloped in performance ritual. One of my songs called "Bledsung" has become an anthem of Judy Grahn's metaformic theory, which, again, posits that the origins of human culture and human consciousness are rooted in menstrual rituals. "Bledsung" highlights some of the many ways our blood rites contribute to what I consider the "blood economy." As a song

of inquiry, *Bledsung* captures in soulful rhythm and jazzy melody
my graduate thesis— *The Men$trual Origins of Money: Radical
Economics in the Presence of the Divine, Sacred Feminine.*

Bledsung
Song Lyrics/Melody by Polly Wood

How come when they say "Man," they mean man, woman, child?
How come when they say "Man," they mean "all people"?

How come they show the blood of Christ,
The blood of war, the blood from the sliced incision
(surgery on t.v. every night)?

How come they show the blood of sport?
It's all the same as blood from violent video games
Movies! They love to see Hollywood stars in a bloody fight.

How come they drink the blood of life
As red wine, buy the bloody meat from the butcher's vine?
It's all accepted, all okay

Except the blood they cannot say
Except the blood you cannot say
Except the blood you cannot speak
Except that blood may sometimes leak.

The only blood they cannot show
Is the blood that freely, freely flows
From ladies, sisters, women, girls, and me.

No cut, no scrape, no knife, no gun, no wound.
No cut, no scrape, no knife, no gun, no wound.
No cut, no scrape, no knife, no gun, no wound.

Well it flowed before hunting, it flowed before time.
Our blood revealed the gift that is the human mind.
Now it's bloodshed for profit, they treat blood like gold.

They've created a blood debt and our families are sold.

They advertise, they televise the violence and the lies.
The violence, the lies.
And it's all accepted, all okay,

Except the blood they cannot say
Except the blood you cannot say
Except the blood you cannot speak
Except that blood may sometimes leak.

The only blood they cannot show
Is the blood that freely, freely flows
From ladies, sisters, women, girls, and me.

Its how we came to be, oh, menstrual-lunar synchrony.
Its how we came to be, oh, Metaformic Theory.

No cut, no scrape, no knife, no gun, no wound.
No cut, no scrape, no knife, no gun, no wound.
No cut, no scrape, no knife, no gun, no wound.

Its how we came to be, oh, it's how we came to be.
Its how we came to be, oh, it's how we came to be.

ON SEEING WITH THE MENSTRUAL MIND

My thesis explores the intersection of two main theories: metaformic theory and economic theory. As a creative woman who was continually questioning my own worth and the value of what I had to offer the world, I discovered that the extraordinary yet common blood rites that informed my life—and that were clearly essential to the wellbeing of our human culture—had no measurable value in our global economic system. Somehow, I had internalized this lack of monetary value as a personal lack of self-worth. I realized that this free-flowing blood and its ability to create and carry new life were being suppressed through the global economic system, which attempted to erase its inherent value. This system of measurement is at the foundation of those who create public policy to protect and preserve what is considered valuable. If women's blood rites are not valued by that system, they will not be protected by that system. They, in fact, could be exploited instead of being honoured and preserved.

As Grahn states in the in the foreword to her book *Blood, Bread, and Roses: How Menstruation Created the World*, "Cross-culturally, ethnographers of native cultures have often been told that women's rites hold the world in balance" (xi). Yet these rites, and the power contained in women's bloodshed in the free-flowing blood of menstruation—the only blood that is not traumatically induced—are considered taboo. In the majority of our global communities, women's blood is hidden away or visually represented by blue liquid. Industrialized, First-World countries create and promote products that assist in the hiding of this sacred blood. With so many options for how to hide menstrual blood, nearly half of the world's population will, at some point, have the potential to internalize the shaming message that our global economy gives: menstrual blood has no value and should not be seen.

According to metaformic theory, human consciousness emerged out of carefully managed menstrual seclusion rituals, and the ability to count and keep time in the human mind was born from rituals that marked menstrual-lunar synchrony. Grahn's theory inspires us to see that words such as "measure" and "menstrual" share roots with words meaning "moon," "blood," and "mind." Likewise, the root of the word *"time"* comes from the Proto-Indo-European word *"di-mon,"* meaning "to cut the moon" (Harper). Although the ritual bloodshed of war is commonly used to measure time in global history, our ability to count and measure came from the original bloodshed rituals, from marking cycles of menstruation.

If we think of ritual in terms of the everyday actions of our lives, we can see how the repetition of these actions keeps the order of things while creating meaning. As I have written elsewhere: "Even the history and use of our words are rituals, such as his-story, which, when reenacted, define a system of belief. If the use of our words changes, which they have, and will, the way we function in use of them, as a culture, changes" (22). Ritual has the ability to transform, on an individual level, one's own understanding of the world, and ritual is also the key to social and cultural order and development (Wood 20).

Robbie E. Davis-Floyd—a cultural anthropologist specializing in medical, ritual, and gender studies, and the anthropology of reproduction—states in her book *Birth as an American Rite of Passage*, "Ritual mediates between cognition and chaos by making reality appear to conform to accepted cognitive categories. In other words, to perform a ritual in the face of chaos is to restore conceptual order" (13). Furthermore, she states, "Because the belief system of a culture is enacted through ritual, analysis of ritual can lead directly to a profound understanding of that belief system" (10). If we look at the counting rituals that make up our global accounting system, and how they recognize bloodshed, we will gain an understanding of the belief system that our economy values.

THE ECONOMICS OF WELLBEING

How do we care for what is sacred to us? How do we measure what we find valuable? If things we value are not counted in the current economic system, how can we respond, personally and collectively, to acknowledge their presence and protect them if necessary? What alternative means can we use to measure the wellbeing of our world? Seeking to gain more internal calm in the face of a world that continually makes me question my own value and question the value of the things I believe make life worth living, I began creatively inquiring into these questions as a regular practice.

My interest in global economics was inspired by the work of Marilyn Waring, a New Zealand economist who demystified the systems by which all nations measure their country's economic "wellbeing." As the first woman voted into New Zealand's Parliament in the 1970s at the young age of twenty-two, she mastered what she called "the art of the dumb question," specifically questioning the national accounts systems. Through her nine years in Parliament, as chairwoman of the Public Expenditure Select (Public Accounts and Budget) Committee, she asked questions again and again that no one else dared to ask. She asked why the natural environment, subsistence production, the unpaid work and reproductive work of women, and care-based work—whether for children, elderly, or the sick—were not accounted for in her nation's budget.

Waring's work uncovering the economic absurdity of her own country led her around the world in search of a different budgetary model. She discovered that what was being counted (or valued) and not counted (or not valued) was the same for all nations functioning under the United Nations. They measured their country's economic wealth through a uniform accounting system adopted in the 1940s, which, to this day, is the basis of all national accounting. This system became known as the United Nations System of National Accounts (UNSNA) and was developed to measure *the national income of a country at war* (Waring, 44).

The UNSNA measures a country's wellbeing through economic growth. Yet the only things that can be measured are things that can pass through the market. Waring brought to light the fact that the United Nations member nations could only recognize currency changing hands (Wood 38). Those things that do not pass through the market—however peaceful, beautiful, life giving, or life sustaining they may be—cannot be measured and therefore have no value in the global economy. Our world's natural resources in-themselves have no economic value and are not accounted for in the UNSNA, rendering them easily destroyable. Acts of destruction, however, such as a giant oil spill in our ocean or the clear cutting of ancient trees, are actually accounted for as an increase to the economy's growth. As Waring writes:

> The current state of the world is the result of a system that attributes little or no "value" to peace. It pays no heed to the preservation of natural resources or to the labour of the majority of its inhabitants or to the unpaid work of the reproduction of human life itself—as well as its maintenance and care. *The system cannot respond to values it refuses to recognize.* (3)

Waring's work exposes that what is counted as economically "productive" has measurable value. Those things contribute to the wellbeing and growth of our global economy. What cannot pass through the market is not considered economically productive, is not accounted for, and has no measurable value. Unfortunately, much of what contributes to economic growth comes at the expense of human lives; it destroys cultures, natural resources, and true wellbeing. Such is the fate of the placenta, the amazing organ, without which, life for us would be impossible. Placentas will continue to be considered worthless unless we reclaim them as powerful reminders of our peaceful and valuable blood rituals.

METAFORMIC ECONOMICS

Metaformic economics locates women's sacred blood power at the centre of life; it creates and sustains cultural rituals that honour this blood. Otherwise, the act of hiding women's blood power or treating it as waste adds to the profit-driven economy of a country through the production, sale, and consumption of all the products that keep this blood hidden. Mass advertising efforts about these products promote and propagate the message that women's blood, including placenta and lochial blood, should not be seen. As Jordan writes, "In the exchange economy, value only becomes apparent when the market assigns it to the placenta, which comes in the form of stem cell research, as well as cosmetics industry uses of placentas" (282). Likewise, a childbearing woman who becomes medically managed through the technocratic model of maternity care offered by modern medicine increases the wealth of a nation. The UNSNA has no way to measure the value of women's blood for its life-giving properties but measures profit from the shame of its hidden nature. By creating profit-driven rituals around women's bloodshed, the inherent value is stripped away from the source and is given to those who create and sell the products that hide it. This includes the professionals who manage birth and the technology employed in its management.

The blood of war also increases the wealth of a nation. War requires intentional acts of violent bloodshed and is both glorified and valued as economically productive. The same goes for the violent blood that is seen in film, television, video games, and violent sporting events. Metaformic theory, says Judy Grahn, "goes directly to the roots of what has been most sacred for human beings" (*Are Goddesses* 1). By looking at the incessant, mass, violent ritual bloodshed of our world with a metaformic mind, one would think that *this* is the blood that we hold sacred.

If we look to the roots of the word "economics," we'll see that it comes from the Latin *"oikonomikos"* meaning "the care and management of a household" (Waring 15). If we expand our thinking of "household" to mean "home," and in the greatest sense "Earth" as our global community's home, we can view the roots of economics to mean how we care for and manage our home, our communities, our planet. Economics, at its root, is not about money but is about *how we care for and manage that which is sacred to us.* Far from the roots of the word itself, we can see that our current economy is based on a skewed system of measurement, and it is up to us to find creative ways to protect and preserve what we consider valuable.

CONCLUSION

For land mammals, when conception occurs, the menstrual blood stops flowing and the placenta begins to form. Without the placenta, there would be no land mammals, including our own human species. Besides humans and camels, all land mammals—including animals of prey, predators, carnivores, and herbivores—eat their placenta after giving birth. For human mammals in the modern world, "placentophagy," or the act of ingesting the placenta, is a relatively new thing, although the placenta has been used as a remedy in traditional Chinese medicine for centuries. Ethnographic accounts can be found of cultures that cook and eat their placenta in a ritual meal, and many parents bury the placenta as a meaningful act. The placenta is the only organ that is created when it is needed, then expelled when it has completed its function in the womb. In this way, the placentas are a "gift," as Nané speaks of in "A Poetics of the Placenta." They can even be a double gift of sorts: first gifting life to a new baby, then giving nourishment to the mammalian mothers who ingest them. We care for the placenta because it is sacred and because it is a valuable gift.

Placentas are extraordinary organs, and for a mother to save her placenta from hazardous waste in today's blood economy is a revolutionary act. For a mother to choose to honour her placenta in whatever way she sees fit gives value to the life-giving power of our blood. By valuing our bloody placentas, we disrupt the economic status quo and we highlight the consciousness-bringing and life-affirming roots of economics, of how we care for what is truly sacred to us.

WORKS CITED

Davis-Floyd, Robbie E. *Birth as an American Rite of Passage.* University of California Press, 1992.

Grahn, Judy. *Blood, Bread, and Roses: How Menstruation Created the World.* Beacon Press, 1993.

Grahn, Judy. *Are Goddesses Metaformic Constructs? An Application of Metaformic Theory to Menarch Celebrations and Goddess Rituals of Kerala and Contiguous States in South India.* Dissertation, California Institute of Integral Studies, 1999.

Harper, Douglas. *Online Etymological Dictionary.* Douglas Harper, 2017, *www.etymonline.com.* Accessed 20 Apr. 2017.

Jordan, Nané. "A Poetics of the Placenta: Placental Cosmology as Gift and Sacred Economy." *She Is Everywhere!: An Anthology of Writing in Womanist/Feminist Spirituality,* edited by Mary Saracino and Mary Beth Moser, vol. 3, IUniverse, 2012, pp. 276-292.

Selander, Jodi. "*Research and Articles.*" *Placenta Remedies Network,* 2017, https://placentaremediesnetwork.org/research-and-articles/. Accessed 20 Apr. 2017.

Waring, Marilyn. *Counting for Nothing—What Men Value and What Women Are Worth.* University of Toronto Press, 1999.

Wood, Polly. *The Men$trual Origins of Money: Radical Economics in the Presence of the Divine, Sacred Feminine.* Lulu Publishing, 2007.

14.
A Placenta by Any Other Name

VALERIE BOREK

The named is the Mother of all things.
—Lao Tzu (*Tao Te Ching*)

I WAS SO HAPPY WITH MY SON'S PLACENTA. My midwife told me it was almost the largest she had ever seen. It was robust, firm, and moist; it was red and purple. I was irrationally and unapologetically proud. But I couldn't articulate why. I didn't yet know how to trust knowledge that cannot be spoken in words. My brain was bound to the rational, where things and people have to be labelled and appraised, and where it is dangerous and threatening to recognize the radical power inherent in the female form.

The placenta is the ultimate protector and nourisher. That is one way I have categorized it. It is a manifestation of the limbic space of transition. It is a facilitator of creation. It is the keystone of a woman's life cycles, symbolized in the blood mysteries. It represents the sacred link between mother and child. I see it as metaphorically my Self, as a powerful creator and healer. But I've gotten ahead of myself. It took time for me to find words to describe my thoughts on the placenta.

What's in a name? That which we call a rose would smell as sweet and that which we call a placenta would still facilitate life, were it not by that name called. Words have power, and a name may be the most powerful type of word because it creates the reality and rules of the thing named. A name shapes perceptions. It is a self-fulfilling prophecy. A rose may retain its perfume no matter its name, but if we call that thorny bush an invasive weed, its fragrance has a different fate than if the petals are "prize winning." With a name, we label, we categorize, and we create. And what we create, we control—or do we?

My reverence for the placenta started simply by following a compelling question—why has such a powerful organ been marginalized by institutions we tend to see as authoritative, such as in medicine and law? In this essay, I'll take you on my journey to answer these questions. In the coming pages, you'll read the story of a mother's legal battle for her right to retain her placenta for encapsulation (*printed in italics*), in which I was involved as an attorney. That story entwines with my own experience with the placenta—as an attorney, as a mother, and as a woman.

WHO OWNS A PLACENTA?

Early one morning, I got a call I wasn't expecting. A local midwife transferred a client from home to hospital, where Mom had a successful birth. "But she may need an attorney" the midwife warned, "because the hospital won't let her have her placenta." I was stunned. I was a new mother and a young attorney. I was naïve. What kind of people would simply claim a part of someone else's body? Someone else's birth right? Of course. I would help.

Who owns a placenta? It depends. (Lawyers love saying that.) The name assigned by the people you ask foreshadows the fate:

What are you going to do with your afterbirth?
What are you going to do with your baby's spiritual twin?
What are you going to do with that medical waste?
What are you going to do with those human remains?

It becomes clear that the label used is determinative. Mothers and midwives use different terms than doctors and lawyers to describe a placenta. After a home birth or at a respectful institution, Mom decides whether the placenta is encapsulated, buried, immortalized as art, none of the above, or a little of all. Doctors and lawyers use terms like refuse, remains, tissue, organ, and medical waste. Each medico-legal term implies valuation, ownership, and control by an interloper in the sacred process of birth.

Once a mom walks into a hospital, she is subject to their rules. In medicalized birth, a hierarchy of rules and labels are applied to a woman's body, her baby, and her birth experience. In order of descending authority, these are the following: federal and state law, agency regulation, hospital policy, and provider preference (influenced by professional societies and perceived risk of litigation). Hence, doctors face a matrix of overlapping rules, fears, and risk factors that influence their practice. Note that mother's wishes aren't on the list.

These rules have serious consequences for labouring women. Moms face protocols and policies that dictate procedures, which can cascade into more procedures. Society's rules then demand homage for "saving" Mom or the baby from conditions that might have been nonexistent without interventions. These interventions surely can be lifesaving when deployed during a medical emergency. However, in general in the U.S., during birth, doctors save mothers from the natural process of their bodies. After birth, mothers are further saved from their placentas.

I called the new mother at the hospital. She was merely a few hours postpartum, but her adrenaline was high. She wanted to encapsulate her baby's placenta. The new mother told the staff she was getting a lawyer and demanded the placenta be preserved on ice. Astutely, she spoke the only language the medico-legal system understands—the threat of economic consequences through litigation.

As of 2016, only three states explicitly protect the right to take home a placenta: Hawaii, Oregon, and Texas. In all other states the law is silent, leaving disposition to the whim of local rules and provider preference. Most American women have no desire to see or use their placenta, but this is changing. More and more women are drawn to use the placenta in their own way, according to their instincts, but they are finding the law is not generally on their side.

The right to privacy and autonomy over one's body is so strong in the United States that it resonates even after death. It is one of the few countries where citizens must actively elect organ donation. Americans are shocked when they learn that they do not have absolute property rights in their bodies. So why do we have such a conflict over the placenta? Shouldn't the disposition automatically be at the discretion of the individual?

There was no law protecting the mom's right to her baby's placenta, so the hospital was calling the shots. Their policy was to send placentas to the pathology lab for destruction because they were identified as medical waste. At first, Mom was simply told her placenta was off limits. But lawyers have more clout than mothers when the bottom line is on the line. Once I began a conversation with hospital counsel, I was told mom could have her placenta only if it was rendered biologically safe with formaldehyde. Clearly, this was not an option for a Mom who wanted to ingest through encapsulation. But the hospital's position had moved, so I hoped. I felt fiercely protective of this hostage placenta, as I did with my own son's, when he was born months before.

BIRTH CHOICES

When I became pregnant, I chose home birth with the nonchalant arrogance of an American. It never even crossed my mind that my decision wouldn't be fully enabled and supported by law. I thought I lived in the land of the free and home of the brave. I quickly learned that in the United States homebirth is a radical choice. I never would have believed I'd have an unlicensed provider attend my birth, but that is the sorry state of the law where I live. I experienced shock after shock at how my choice to birth at home was villainized by health providers, feared by family and friends, and—the deepest cut to my heart—challenged by the law. I could understand human ignorance, but how could an institution meant to protect our rights, instead actively suppress them? This was the very institution I entrenched myself in, because I believed it to be a bastion of justice and fairness from which I could protect the freedom I hold so dearly. My inner Lady Justice stirred.

My partner wanted to know if I would eat the placenta. He proudly showed me videos of dutiful men making placenta smoothies, scrambled eggs, and sautés. I had never given one thought to the afterbirth. Now I was supposed to eat it with my eggs? I considered myself open minded, but this was one realm of hippie motherhood I was not ready to embrace. Yet I was intrigued. I wondered: why do people do that? What's the benefit? What power can be drawn from this organ?

To help the mother with the hostage placenta, I realized I just needed to go to the source of the power. Who was the creator in the world of labels, laws, money, and medicine? The Department of Health defined medical waste, organs, tissues, and blood products in legal terms but was silent on placentas. According to law, the hospital was not prevented from releasing the afterbirth, provided public health would not be at risk. It turned out the only hang-up was the name the hospital chose to give the placenta: "medical waste." In using that label, the hospital invoked rules of disposal. Had the hospital called the placenta an "organ" instead, for example, it would not have triggered the procedure being used. Facing the threat of a court action, a black mark on their marketing, and now armed with knowledge there would be no penalty from the state, the hospital did their math and agreed to let Mom have her frozen, unpreserved placenta. It would cost them less—provided she sign a release of liability, of course.

PONDERING THE PLACENTA: SEEDING THE DIVINE FEMININE

Legal and scientific fascination with the placenta ultimately helped me reclaim my birth rights and rites as a woman. My curiosity of the biology and history of the placenta seeded my spiritual awakening, creeping and embedding into my heart like organic villi. Pondering the placenta was my gateway to the divine feminine. This latter term needs definition because it means so much to so many, and it is probably not what you think. At first, the divine feminine wasn't anything I could conceive. As a child, I rejected the concept of "female" that was presented to me. I hated pink and refused dresses. I also rejected feminism of the day.

I never understood why a movement centered on women's empowerment left such a bad taste in my mouth. I finally realized it was because women were fighting to be like men—to be "daughters of the father." Women fought to assert their worth and power in a world that was not theirs, and the fight to justify the right to participate eclipsed actual BE-ing. It was the fight itself that I now know felt wrong to me. Women pushed against a glass ceiling in an economic system never meant to honour the simplicity of existing and nurturing life (Wood). I feel it is the essence of the feminine not to assimilate but to transform and transcend.

I do not see the divine or the sacred feminine in this form of feminism. True female empowerment is recognizing the value and power of the female's contribution to life, independent of values that we hold so dearly in society today—those of hyper-rationality and commerce, to be specific. The essence of the feminine force in the universe has inherent value and power. It is the antithesis of this dominating rationality and commodification that is central to our world today. The feminine sparks an internal process, not external control. It is power with, not power over (Starhawk). The sacred feminine energy is like the placenta—nourishing, protecting, and healing all life, for the purpose of growth.

When I was a child, like most girls, I didn't question my mother when she told me it was time for The Pill. I embraced it, buying into the thought it gave me control over my body. I never questioned whether my body should be controlled. It was a great idea, since I thought I never wanted to become a mother. I was focused on earning success through hard work. All of this changed when I chose to stop birth control, but not for the reasons you may be thinking.

I stopped ingesting hormones for the first time in almost twenty years after recognizing a link between my mental state and the medication. I had been mildly but chronically depressed for some time, but things took a turn for the worse when the economy tanked at the same time I was graduating from law school. Being unemployed, perpetually justifying my self and capabilities through interview after interview, can definitely wreak havoc on self-esteem and lead to some serious questions. Who am I really?

As my depression grew deeper, I started grasping at ways to stop the slide. I saw that my emotional stability was affected by different doses and brands of hormones. So I chose to stop. Once I stopped the routine of the pill, my mental state shifted. I started seeing things differently. I was feeling things more. I made a huge leap and decided to start a family.

After the birth of my son, I chose the only option for birth control that I knew of without hormones—an IUD. My instinct was crying out for me to find a different way. But in the overwhelming blur of new motherhood, I relented. What choice did I have?

My body erupted into conditions that seemed to come out of the blue. The depression that had been constant, like static in the background from a radio dial not properly tuned, blew up into serious postpartum depression. I raged. My monthly cycles were frequent and heavy. I had dry eye. I finally listened to my inner being after a transient cyst screamed at me that something was terribly wrong in the lady-parts department. I had the IUD removed and almost instantaneously the issues resolved themselves. Through this experience, I found confidence in listening to my instinct that cannot always be expressed in words, and doesn't need a peer-reviewed study to justify its truth.

I found natural family planning and slowly started reconnecting with my body. I started feeling more grounded. Unwittingly, I had started a journey back to who I was ... the *me* I didn't know was lost. It was a beautiful and difficult journey. I was on a quest to find my true power, although I did not yet understand what the divine feminine can gift us. I remember telling my sister that in becoming a mother, I no longer had the luxury of ignoring my mental baggage.

They say the road to hell is paved with the best intentions. I had intentions of practising law as if it were a healing art. I wanted to help people heal their wounds through the mechanism of the legal system. However, in only three short years after helping with the hostage placenta, I witnessed injustice over and over again, especially with respect to women and the sacred. There are occasional victories, as there was for this new mom, but it isn't enough, and it is not going to change. I thought I would be able to help people by wielding the sword of Lady Justice, but I now see that the structure in place is not geared toward healing. Just as I rejected feminism for pushing against the current, I am transcending the legal system in favour of searching for a way to create healing by working with the flow of energy. That is truly the essence of justice that the Lady stands for. The system doesn't need to be changed, any more than a tiger needs new stripes. Courts aren't made for healing, and no amount of money can buy true justice in the way it resonates with the heart. Lady Justice was welcomed into the court room as a mollifying gesture. She never belonged there, and neither do I. Becoming an attorney was a trial I had to undergo to begin to understand that true justice and healing must begin with the self.

DESCENT AND PLACENTAL POWER

There is a myth of a Sumerian goddess named Inanna, Queen of Heaven and Earth (Brinton Perera). In one story, she descends to the underworld to visit her sister, the dark and violent Ereshkegal, who grieves the death of her husband. Along the way, Inanna has to shed her attire and regalia, and ultimately face her sister naked and unadorned. In a rage, Ereshkegal kills her and hangs her corpse from a hook (every family has its problems). There, Inanna stays until she is rescued by spirits sent by a loyal friend. The spirits heal the pain of Ereshkegal by listening to her grief. After being truly heard and seen by these spirits, the Queen of the Underworld releases her hold on her sister and allows Inanna to return to the light.

Surrendering to the birth of goddess consciousness requires one to journey into the dark, like a descent into the underworld. My fascination with the placenta opened that portal. In studying the legal rights a person should have to their placenta, I learned of spiritual practices surrounding birth and the cycles of a woman. As a new mother considering what I would do with this spiritual twin, I learned about the organ and its ability to protect and heal. I wondered how the biology resonated on a spiritual level. I yearned for understanding. What does it mean to have a female form? What can birth teach us about spirituality? How does menstruation become a spiritual practice, and what role could the placenta have in these blood mysteries?

As I delved into learning why the placenta was sacred to so many, I kept coming across the concept of women reclaiming their power. What power? I felt as naked and in the dark as Inanna before Ereshkegal. There were so many points in my life where

I felt powerless—in relationships, in my career, in my own skin. I was always pushing against something, and I felt as if I were losing ground.

In becoming a mother, I was compelled to question the concept of creation of the self and the role the mother plays in nurturing ego in her children. The role is inescapable. A mother will shape her child whether she is conscious of her power or not. Her perception of the world filters the child's understanding, which can help or harm. I realized I had to face myself and take responsibility for the power that I accepted as a mother to help shape my children's concept of themselves and reality.

The biologic role of the placenta in protecting life resonated for me. I was surprised to learn that it protects and heals not just the child but also the mother. It is saturated with stem cells, the cells that generate endless possibilities for creation. I saw with new eyes the strained relationship that I have with my own mother. I never felt close with her. Her parenting style was to protect me by causing me to fear consequences or my own ability to take risks. She loved me in her own way, and wanted to teach me to be an independent woman. However, a life lived in fear is a life of estrangement and disempowerment, and that is especially potent when the fear comes from your mother. Symbolically, a mother is everyone's most tangible manifestation of the divine, as her womb is our gateway from source energy to substance here on earth. So when we feel disconnected from our mothers, we feel disconnected from everything—from life itself, from spirit, from ourselves.

I don't blame my mother for my fears anymore. I've done the work to release that. I've forgiven her, although in retrospect it seems silly to feel the need to forgive someone for simply being who they are. Perhaps I have forgiven the circumstances that kept my mother so distant from me. After all, "The woman I needed to call my mother was silenced before I was born" (Rich 228). Her own fears and suppressed expression are a result of systemic disrespect for sacred feminine principals.

Through my work with the divine feminine, I started envisioning my ability to interrupt the transmission of estrangement to younger generations. I can create a new reality for my blood line. I can create a new heritage based in joy and love rather than fear. And just as a placenta will heal both mother and child, so can I work up and down the matrilineal line by healing myself.

Thus, it was the placenta, my spiritual twin, which rescued me from my own decent into darkness. As I awakened to the sacred feminine, I slowly began shedding all the rules and fears and structures I picked up on my path as a liberated, educated, nurturing woman. I started by abandoning medical management of my monthly blood and didn't stop until I dismantled everything I had known to be true. I chose to let go of everything that wasn't serving me. I cleared my calendar. I closed my law firm. I questioned every relationship and drifted away from those that were not healthy. I made the radical choice to stop trying to make my life happen, and instead just be present and surrender to life itself. The first steps were like moving mountains, but I am now running like an avalanche down that mountain back to the self I had lost.

My study of the placenta nourished my soul enough to make me realize the power of the feminine is the power to create. To shape reality. To give form. To nurture and heal and sustain life. I started to understand this is the inherent power in the womb. Creation, and thus healing, is the power of the divine feminine.

I realized that the placenta has eluded commodification, and for that reason, its inherent value has been ignored by science and, in turn, the law. Its inherent power cannot be commodified because it is the power we all have inside of us as our birthright. This "flat cake," as it was known to the Greeks, cannot be revered in a social framework like our commercial culture, which demands a person look outside herself for happiness and healing. If it cannot be commodified, it must be marginalized in our socioeconomic terms.

The placenta is power with, not power over. It is creation, not domination. It is love and acceptance, not fear and estrangement. Understanding this basic concept has opened doors in my life. It has made me realize that I can consciously create my life anew.

So what's in a name?

Creation. And that is exactly what the placenta is: the power of creation, transformation, and healing.

One man's medical waste is another woman's treasure.
WORKS CITED

Brinton Perera, Sylvia. *Descent to the Goddess.* Inner City Books, 1981.

Laozi. *Tao Te Ching: A New English Version.* Edited by Stephen Mitchell, Harper & Row, 1988.

Rich, Adrienne. *Poems: Selected and New, 1950-1974.* WW Norton & Company, 1980.

Starhawk. *Dreaming the Dark: Magic, Sex and Politics.* Beacon Press, 1997.

Wood, Polly. *The Menstrual Origins of Money: Radical Economics in the Presence of The Divine, Sacred Feminine.* Lulu Publishing, 2007.

15.
"Baby's Life Is in the Placenta Only"

Hearing Dais' Voices in India

JANET CHAWLA

HAVING GIVEN BIRTH TO THREE CHILDREN and being the proud grandmother of five, I know a bit about the placenta—should I say from a user's point of view? But that doesn't exactly qualify me to write this paper. Rather it is my involvement with birthing mothers for over forty years—first as leader of exercise classes for pregnant women in Oakland and San Francisco, California, then as a teacher of birth preparation classes in New Delhi, India, and then as an educator doing orientations about natural childbirth or nonmedicalized birth in many states of India—that qualifies me. Most recently, I have founded a non-governmental organization called MATRIKA, and have worked as an ethnographer researcher for the Jeeva Research Project. Both of these groups value the contributions of "dais," or Indigenous Indian midwives, to the wellbeing of poor and rural women, and perceive their skills and rituals to be relevant to all birthing mothers. Much of this paper will be drawn from research done by the Jeeva Project, which conveys the words and experiences of the dais themselves.

First, I would like to mention that one of India's earliest texts, the *Atharva Veda*, includes this religio-medical incantation about a birth and a placenta:

> At this birth ... let the woman rightly engender, may her joints relax, that she shall bring forth! ... loosen the womb ... let go the embryo!

> Attached not at all to the flesh, nor to the fat, not at all

190

to the marrow,
may the splotched, moist, placenta come down.... May
the placenta fall down!

I split open thy vagina, thy womb, thy canals; I separate
the mother and the
son, the child along with the placenta. May the placenta
fall down!

As flies the wind, as flies the mind, as fly the winged birds,
so do thou, O
embryo, ten months old, fall along with the placenta! May
the placenta fall
down!

(Chapter four, paragraph 01011, verses 1-6).

DAIS: IN THEIR OWN WORDS

Much of the information in this paper is drawn from data generated
by the Jeeva Research Project, particularly multiple interviews with
dais—traditional midwives or traditional birth attendants. Jeeva
does collaborative, multidisciplinary, and multicentric research on
dais, their childbirth practices, and their public health significance
in four remote sites of India. Jeeva was directed by six researchers from diverse fields: public health, medicine, nurse-midwifery,
natural childbirth, and ethnography. They were collectively called
the "Jeeva Shepherds." The project was hosted and financially
managed by the Centre for Women's Development Studies, New
Delhi, from 2010 to 2015.

The goal of the Jeeva study was to examine the role of experienced dais in their own social context with reference to neonatal
and maternal survival and wellbeing—with a focus on stimulation of the placenta to revive a newborn—and to highlight the
relevance of dais in meeting public health concerns. Underserved
sites were purposely selected where the dai tradition, or remnants
of it, were still active. These areas were in Kangra District of
Himachal Pradesh, Bokharo District of Jharkand, Nandurbar

District of Maharashtra, and Bellary District of Karnataka. We encouraged the local researchers to "actively listen" to what the dais were saying, allowing words and categories to emerge in the data; we made sure that the data was not fitting into researchers' preconceived categories. We also encouraged the local researchers' liberal use of empathy and imagination. Importantly, researchers lived for two years within the communities that they were documenting.

THE POWERFUL PLACENTA

No traditional birth attendant, and here I am using the word "dai" to mean traditional birth attendant, would ever cut the umbilical cord before the placenta was delivered. India is such a varied place, culturally and geographically, and few statements can be made that are true for all peoples across regions and cultural differences. However, not cutting the cord before the placenta is born is true across the length and breadth of the Indian subcontinent. The importance of the connection between placenta and cord to the newborn is known, especially in how to revive the baby when the need arises.

RESUSCITATION

If the baby does not cry, or is limp and seemingly not breathing after birth, then the dais, families, and traditional communities understand that its life has stayed back in the placenta. One dai from Jharkhand explained how the placenta is then used:

I was there when this woman's *bachcha* [infant] was born, and it was completely unconscious. The people of the house started to cry; they all told the woman that 'you have given birth to a dead baby.' She also started crying and then fainted. I saw every part of the *bachcha*'s body. It felt warm, and I could also sense light *phus-phus nikaas* [breath]. Then I asked everybody to stop crying. I put the *phool* [placenta] in warm water and after some time and a lot of effort, the *bachcha* started to cry. But this whole procedure took about three to four hours. Then I could assure the family that the baby was ok. (Burdhi Sahis from Jharkhand)

Dais are adept at drawing upon the normative physiological functioning of the human body and enhancing that functioning in their caregiving. Their work to revive a limp, unconscious (or not), and breathing neonate is an excellent example of the placenta's capacity. Understanding, handling, and valuation of the placenta was common to all dais that were interviewed:

If the child doesn't breathe, then I put the phool in hot water. It should be just hot enough so that my hand can bear it. I rub the cord. When the child cries only then I cut the cord.... In doing all this it takes me one to one and a half hours. If the child still does not cry, then I do not do anything else. Then I understand that child would not survive.... I learned from my elder saas [mother-in-law] how to heat phool. My daadi saas [grandmother-in-law] also used to do the same. (Abola Sahis from Jharkhand)

We take water and pat the placenta. As we pat placenta it becomes blown up. If the placenta moves then the baby will move, it will breathe ... it gives life to the baby through cord and through navel. As air goes inside, then the ribs and sides pulsate, the chest pulsates. It happens we come to know. (Dayamakka from Karnataka)

If the baby is not crying or moving, then we heat an earthen pot, wrap the placenta in a cloth, and put it in that pot. (Dhusari from Himachal Pradesh)

If the baby doesn't cry, then its life goes back into the placenta. When that happens, we have to keep some burning coals on a clay tile. Over that, we give heat to the placenta and pull the life from the kuchru [placenta] through the cord to the baby. I hold the saatli [placenta] with one hand and rub the cord toward the baby with my other hand.

After it cries, we tie a thread around the cord and cut it. (Velki from Maharashtra)

From the retrospective birth survey, another Jeeva interview tool, resuscitation by stimulating the placenta was confirmed by a mother:

It took birth as if it has died, looking like dead. The dai told me that there is life in placenta, so she pressed placenta and while pressing the cord from placenta to child it was not even breathing, but then she sneezed, then cried.

Warmth (*sek*) can be applied to the baby as well as to the placenta for revival:

Healthy baby cries, and weak baby does not. At hospital there is medicine, but at home, all this is not there. At home, *thaali* [steel plate] is banged, splash water on baby, give oil to baby's whole body, head and ears, give *sek* [dry heat] from fire, then baby starts crying. After giving *sek*, put baby next to mother and cover it and make it sleep. That makes baby warm and it starts crying. (Hemkala from Himachal)

Warmth or *sek* is also mentioned as a component of the 'life' flowing to the baby while milking the cord:

If the baby doesn't cry then I milk the *naal* [cord] slowly toward the baby. It brings warmth into the baby's body, and it starts crying. (Bhadu from Jharkhand)

Baby's life remains in the placenta. When baby doesn't cry, then I first give *sek* from the fire to the baby. Then I put *phool* in hot water. Baby starts crying. (Abola from Jharkhand)

In Karnataka, in Southern India, cold water is used for resuscitation:

If the baby is lying without crying, then the placenta is

put in cold water, and baby is kept there, and a glass of
cold water and then hot water are put over its chest alternatively and patted; the person standing by the side will
take a pounding stick and beat the floor beside the baby or
placenta softly. We chant "give life oh mother, give life oh
mother," then life comes slowly. (Vali Bai from Karnataka)

In all areas, other methods, besides using the placenta for revival, were also mentioned. Dais stated that the need to revive or
resuscitate was not that common among the births they attended.
All procedures involved some kind of stimulation to "awaken" the
baby. Methods used were the following: blowing in ear or mouth;
splashing baby with water; beating a plate or drum with a stick;
slapping, especially of feet; massaging baby; turning baby upside
down; and checking that the mouth clear.

It was also understood that revival was often necessary because
of difficulties the newborn encountered in the birth process—either
the cord or placenta or baby was pressed in such a way that life
and breath were not reaching the infant. This resulted in a "blue,"
limp, or seemingly lifeless baby, as in described here: "Baby gets
stuck in the path, then baby gets pressed and does not cry after
the birth. It cannot breathe. Then I don't cut the cord. There is air
in the cord and so the baby can breathe with it."

Some dais reported a sense of warmth or slight movement in
either the placenta or baby, so were reluctant to pronounce the
newborn as "dead," even though family members had already
begun to wail. A few dais admitted that sometimes, despite trying
to revive, the newborn did not live. A few said that if the fetus had
died in the womb, it could not be revived.

The retrospective birth survey interviewed mothers who had
recently given birth and confirmed much of the dais' interview
statements:

Just after the birth the child did not cry. The dai sprinkled
water on the child's face, but it did not cry. Then she dipped
the placenta in hot water, and slowly she started to pull
the cord toward the child. After repeating this for some
time, the child started crying.

The grandmother of the respondent said that after the delivery the baby did not cry. Then she sprinkled water on the face of the child and banged the plate. Even then when the baby did not cry, the placenta was dipped in lukewarm water and massaged with fingers. Then only the baby got life and cried.

Researchers also heard about the wellbeing of infants revived in this way and heard of no problems with these children later in their lives:

Many years ago I revived a baby by heating her *phool*. Now she is grown up and married too. (Kunti Sahis from Jharkhand)

When the baby doesn't cry, still there is some life in it, even if most of the life has gone back into the *kuchru* [placenta].... Three years ago, I heated the *kuchru* of Foparya's daughter-in-law. The baby was born soon but did not cry. The family members started crying and I told them to be calm. I heated the *kuchru* for a short time and the baby started moving. That was a baby boy, and he is three years old now. They stay in this village. (Makya from Maharashtra)

Humour occasionally enters narrative descriptions: "I have not performed any delivery where the baby was not breathing. Problems urinating and all such cases I have not seen. After delivery it urinates on us only" (JayaBai from Karnataka).

A dais in Jharkhand also shared that the cord will reveal something about this woman's future childbearing. The effects of spousal violence are also mentioned in this passage:

Placenta will be dark and black to see. It will be like a goat's. There will be small knots. We come to know more children are there.... Placenta doesn't tear into pieces. It will be broad. If the person is big, then placenta will also be big. It will not become torn to pieces. If the husband hits the stomach, then danger will be there. (Mallamma from Karnataka)

Placenta is like 'mutton.' It will be round. It will be red. It will not be broken. For some, it will be strong, for some it will be big; it depends on the person's strength. (Phirmabhi from Karnataka)

The placenta and afterbirth are bloody and messy—biomedical institutions consider it to be garbage, unneeded, and only to be disposed of. But dais handle this organ with respect and use its power. Traditionally oriented families share in these notions of placenta power and often bury it with respect. In the traditional mindset, no distinctions between religion and medicine exist, as displayed in the childbirth religio-medical incantation in the Atharva Veda, quoted above.

IMAGE IDIOMS FOR PLACENTA: *PHUL* AND *PHOOL*

In Delhi, Jharkhand, Uttar Pradesh and other places, the placenta is termed the *phool* (the flower), and the baby is the *phul* (the fruit)—an analogy drawn from processes of the natural world. The placenta is, therefore, called the *phool*. As one dai explained, "The *phool* helps the child to breathe. For example inside a person's body or even inside a tree there is *jaan* [life]. If I am healthy and strong, then so is the *phool*. If the *phool* is not there, then there is nothing" (Manji from Jhakhand).

During research in Nandurbar district of Maharashtra I was uncomfortable with what was coming out of our data transcripts, where the only word for placenta was *kachroo*, which refers to what needs "to be thrown away." A tribal woman then said there was another, older word for placenta, *saataro*, which literally means "beehive." It is interesting to understand the placenta as a beehive—making honey (making baby) —or as being a site of growth and communal activity, like the beehive. Also, the little segments of a beehive resemble the cotyledons of the maternal side of the placenta, which are small, interconnecting, lobelike formations.

NARAK

The dais, especially in Jharkhand, sometimes speak of the placenta and afterbirth as *"narak kund."* Although it is often translated as "hell" or a demonic place, *narak* can be better understood as the site or energy of the unseen, the inner world of the earth and the body. What we call "pollution taboos" are related to *narak*. In the orthodox religious traditions, what is considered "sacred" is separated from women's menstrual blood and postpartum blood, also called lochia. Sacred texts from Leviticus of the Old Testament of the Bible to the *Shastras* of the Hindu traditions consider women unclean at these times of bleeding.

I first learned of the dais' understanding of *narak* about twenty years ago, during our MATRIKA research project. The team was sitting on my drawing room floor, mulling over how to translate the phrase *"nau mahene ka narak kund,"* or "nine month's hellish pond," that is used by the dais to signify the afterbirth and the combination of placenta, cord, and amniotic sac. We knew we were not dealing with the Christian "fire and brimstone" hell, the abode of the damned. But even the Hindi word *"narak"* is translated into English as "hell," with very negative associations. We were discussing what exactly a *"kund"* was and how to translate that into English. It was said to be a spring-fed body of water, which had no streams running into it, but water that pulsates up through the earth. As I moved my hand upside down, fingers pointing up to demonstrate the pulsation movement, I realized that the same gesturing had been used by one of my childbirth education instructors to demonstrate the functioning of the placenta. *Kund* is another example of the parallel between nature and the mother's body.

Obviously, dais speak differently from pundits or Hindu priests about the meaning of *narak*. Our MATRIKA team came to think of it as "the open body," which is normally closed. Yet at the time of menstruation and postbirth, the woman's bleeding body is open: "Girls are considered holy before puberty. The marriage of a young girl, who has not had her periods, is performed with her sitting on her father's lap. After puberty the woman is considered unclean, and is unholy, because she bleeds, and this is Narak" (Satya Devi, Bihar).

In another sense, the time of *narak* is marked by what we call "pollution" taboos or ritual uncleanness. Women cannot perform tasks requiring cleanliness, like cooking or entering the kitchen, nor can they perform any kind of religious or prayer activities:

> On *Chatti* day [the sixth day after birth], the *narak* period ends. The dai checks if the umbilical cord has fallen off. Then she bathes the baby and beats a *thaali* [plate]. After this, the woman is bathed and wears new clothes. The dai cleans the room where the delivery took place, and the woman was kept separately for six days. The dirty clothes of mother and child are washed. After this, the dai is given soap and oil for bathing. All this is on the sixth day after delivery. (Kanta, Bihar)

Narak then has many simultaneous meanings for the dais. In one sense, it is the site of unseen inner world of earth and body. From the dominant perspective, it is filthy, bloody, and polluted. As Kamla said, "I can handle *narak*, I don't feel repulsion." This is a time that is out of normal social control, within the terrain of the generative processes of women's lives, within which the dai is empowered to negotiate. Such cycles are differentiated from the world of men and male activities. The term *"narak"* actually encodes deeper notions of the sacredness of fertility in both the earth and women, and in the vulnerability of openness in female cycles, such as menstruation and birth giving. The withdrawal from everyday activities during menses and postpartum could be viewed as a time for much needed rest and renewal in the work of women's lives.

PLACENTAS ASSIST CONCEPTION

Whereas the placenta is used to resuscitate a seemingly lifeless newborn, it is also described as facilitating conception of a sup-posedly "barren" woman:

> If a woman is not having a child, sometimes she may be given to hold the newborn of a newly delivered mother while the baby is still attached to the placenta. They give her to hold both the *phal* and the *phool*. After my oldest

daughter, I didn't have another child for seven years. Then my sister-in-law had a child, and my mother-in-law told me to take this freshly born baby into my lap, and I did so. After this my children started coming again. When it is done like this, that child, who is given in the lap, comes to belong half to the woman who took I in her lap [the term for adoption is "to take in the lap"]. In different castes of people, in this same way, a woman may be allowed to "adopt" the child of another same-caste woman. No one disapproves of this. (Burdi, Jharkhand)

I understand that this ritual of assisted conception draws on the human body's immense and unknown capacities. A woman who takes a neonate and placental mess into her lap immediately after birth will have all of her senses stimulated by the stuff of child-birth. She feels the smells, sounds, touch, sight, and if she kisses the neonate, even the taste. This sense immersion will affect her physically and emotionally. We know that women in the West who have been unable to conceive sometimes do so after adopting and mothering a child. Something changes on all levels, after caring for a child.

PLACENTA BURIAL

Birth and the placenta are part of the richness of our informant's lives. Burdi, a dai in Jharkhand, said the following: "This is the room where all of my children have been born. The placentas of all my children are buried here. We call the womb *koop ghara* [well house] and opening of the womb as *koop muha* [mouth of the well]. And we call the *jagah* [the birth canal] as *bhuiya* [the earth, or the place that baby is born onto the earth]." A kind of richness and embodied belonging are lived in this way of knowing.
In India, the powerful placenta and cord are traditionally consid-ered potent substances that may be misused by bad people, who perform "*jadu tona*" or "black magic," which can harm people. The placenta and cord, and birth itself, are understood as sub-stances and times when the spirit world is active. Dais are, thus, entrusted to negotiate this world and to protect against negative

forces. They are the guardians of fertility. In Jharkhand, they are sometimes called to the marriages of those whose birth they attended, thus passing on the blessings of fertility they carry from attending so many births.

For this reason, the powerful placenta was usually buried to protect it from bad people and also from animals. It was buried with reverence, honouring its life-producing power. From Gita Devi in Jharkhand, we heard the following:

The placenta is offered a fist of grain, two knots of tumeric, sindur, three to five pieces of dub ghaas, hotoki phal, and a flower. And we take out a *shubh dhwani* [auspicious sounds] from our mouth according to Bengali tradition. Then in the same house where the birth has taken place, next to the mother's cot, a hole is dug and the placenta is buried. The hole is filled with earth and plastered over with gobar.

In Jharkhand, repeatedly, we also heard that how the placenta is buried affects the timing of the next child:

While burying the placenta in the earth, if it is buried upside down, with the cord below, that woman would not have more babies. If it is buried with the cord up then again she would have children. The woman who had the baby, if she wishes that her next baby should be born after a gap, then the dai digs the pit in the corner of the room deep till her wrist and then buries the *phool* in that. By doing so, next baby would be conceived late, after a gap. If it is buried in a shallow pit then next baby would be conceived soon and in one or one and a half years, she would get her next baby. (Meera Sahis from Jharkhand)

The traditional birth ways of dais are consummately ecological. The sacred is not separate from the physical, so the "dirty stuff" is not separate from the sacred. The entire cycle of life, including death, is accepted and respected. The placenta is thus buried not only to protect it from animals and black magic but to honour it for the service it has provided in the bringing forth new life. Dais from across India described these burial rituals:

> The placenta cord is buried. We also bury rice, sweets, turmeric and a coin along with it. We pray to Mother Earth to receive the dirty stuff. (Punjab)

> We take a lot of care while burying the placenta. Along with it we bury *kumkum*, money, grain, jaggery and a ring. (Rajasthan)

> When dai buries a placenta in the earth, then family members ask me to offer something to the *phool*, then I offer rice and *doob* grass to *phool*. (Jharkhand)

> Near the house, we dig a pit and put the placenta, horse gram, some seeds, cactus and ragi flour. If some part of this afterbirth is taken away, it will not be good for the baby. It decays there. So we put flour, soil, and then a stone is put over it. (Karnataka)

These ways are changing rapidly as the Indian government, in efforts to save mothers' lives and reduce maternal-infant mortality, has advocated institutional birth for all. I feel that we can all learn from dais' ways and that mothers who need hospitals should be able to avail of them. But, in the meantime, birth at home could be accepted and be more supported. As Seema, a dai from Karnataka, said: "We put the placenta in a pot with betel nut and leaf and one rupee and put the pot in a pit and bury it. It should be covered so no fox or dog will eat it. Now they go to hospital where they throw it and who knows what happens. If home birth takes place then it is buried."

Personally, I have learned much from the traditional ways of birthing, Indian ritual customs, and the knowledge and skills of dais. As a scholar, I also have come to appreciate and value that amazing in-between organ, the placenta, as well as the women who traditionally handle the afterbirth without repulsion and with honor. As one Punjabi dai said: "I am proud of this work. The dai is the medium through which new life comes into this world. God is the doer, but the hands are mine."

WORK CITED

Maurice, Bloomfield, editor and translator. *Atharva Veda: Sacred Books of the East*, vol. 42, Oxford Press, 1897.

16.
Placenta Wit and Chick Lit

A Close Textual Analysis of *The Lost Journals of Sylvia Plath* by Kimberly Knutsen

JUDY E. BATTAGLIA

IN KIMBERLY KNUTSEN'S FIRST NOVEL, *The Lost Journals of Sylvia Plath*, a piece of literary fiction inspired by many "what ifs," the author plays with narration and time to tell a "would-be" story, complete with many "if-then" scenarios. The whole book is a meditation on motherhood and academe, as two lonesome English literature doctoral candidates (Katie and Wilson) fight and love it out over a series of Midwestern semesters. Katie's younger sister, January, becomes a big part of their lives when she comes to live with them because of an unwanted pregnancy. All parties get intimately involved and mixed up with their neighbours, Steven and Lucy. The two are engaged to each other and attend the local community college. In addition to his relationship with Lucy, Steven has a child named Abby.

Metaphors and images of placentas haunt *The Lost Journals of Sylvia Plath* as they do in Plath's own work. Throughout Knutsen's text, the two sisters, Katie and January, become young mothers; both are almost eerily obsessed by images of the afterbirth. They see images of afterbirth appear in airports, rental cars, begonias, pajama bottoms, and blankets. They recall, as reverie, a neighbour's cat eating her placenta after giving birth to her litter of kittens during a pivotal point in Katie and January's shared childhoods. This chapter uses a feminist psychoanalytic lens to examine the ways in which the placenta is depicted in Knutsen's work and how it is evocative of Plath's own complex relationship to the afterbirth. The images of the feminine are universal and ancestral, playing off notions of feminist narratology and Jungian psychoanalysis.

204

This story is about birth; it is also, simultaneously, about birth order. At the beginning of the book, we meet Katie. She is a lonely, disconnected, and somewhat strange PhD candidate in English Literature. Katie is an Oregon transplant attending a large, Midwestern college to complete her degree. Her mother was a hippie, and her father was a yuppiem who was a relatively absent figure in Katie's childhood. Moreover, Katie was repeatedly raped and sodomized by her father's "golfing buddy" from the time she was eight years old until her early adolescence. Finding a good friend in another girl, Katie began spending more time at her new friend's house after school and on the weekends— escaping time at home and with the rapist, who would intrude on her by invading her home space as well as her corporeal body. Katie is described to the reader as a bright, bouncy redhead. This image of redness and its after effects come into play later as stand-ins for the afterbirth itself in the piece.

Readers are introduced to Katie's younger sister January, who was born in August. She is pale skinned, even though her mother is very tan "almost Indian," wherein "almost" is playing on contemporary Native-blood quantum politics and phenol-typical traits (traits that combine nature and nurture). January has jet-black hair that she dyes platinum blonde and chops up because of the request of her bandmate boyfriend, whom she endlessly agonizes over throughout the novel. The naming in the text performs ritualistic significance, almost in the realm of the occult, similar to how Sylvia Plath started seeing the world once she met and married English poet laureate Ted Hughes. January was born into a displaced, changeable, alienated, and at-odds family unit. Her name does not suit her birth month, which shows the readers instead of being an "august" individual her mother saw her as dreamy, brooding, gloomy, and dark.

In this novel, Knutsen tackles many critical themes but does so with good grace and humour as well as with superb stylistic, syntactic, and substantive strategies—particularly employing a feminist narratology. When we examine the ways in which the author plays with time, neighbourhood, the notion of the family as structure, and even the academy in an antihegemonic and anti-patriarchal way, we can see little fissures occurring in the system, giving us hope as readers and as social actors. Moreover, we also see them being reincorporated and interpolated by that same male-dominant power structure, which can depress but also motivate and inspire us. Much like if we were to uncover Plath's lost journals that Hughes might have either hid or destroyed, we could find something under the mulch and mire, "a phoenix, out of the ashes I rise, with my red hair, and I eat men like air" (1960). The redness as theme is important here; it links Katie to Lady Lazurus in Plath's poem and her with blood and afterbirth.

Instances of blood (menstrual, birth, injury), the colour red, and references to Katie's corporeal body serve to remind us that she is centre, close to home, close to truth. At first, it is important because of the narratology of Knutsen's text. Katie and Wilson's young, thin, blonde, neighbour Lucy runs away with January, in part to be with the guys from the band of Jan's past. Katie still looms large in not only the foreground but the background of the story as well. Chapter thirty-two opens with rich description and imagery both of nature and of January's internal mood, thoughts, and feelings:

> Over the woods, across the street from the gas station, curtains of shimmering red light rose and fell in the sky. "What the hell is it?" January said, through a mouthful of chocolate. "Because it's really freaking me out." Although it wasn't. She was too exhausted to care. She felt as if she were underwater. The night was black and close. It smelled, faintly, of skunk. (359)

The red sky functions here as an umbrella, or a child's safe parachute, as it encloses the two women in their cloaks of fantasy and reverie. Katie is already implanted in both their thoughts. For January, Katie is her saviour, a substitute mother whom she hopes will take her baby to raise and allow January to slip away into an altered state of consciousness. This foggy state of consciousness is suggested by the faint odour of skunk emanating from the cloistered air around the two women. The imagery can be either an actual skunk because they are in the wild, the "over the river and through the woods" time and place of nostalgic story tales, or it could be the pungent stench of marijuana. This would foreshadow Lucy and January's soon-to-be altered states of awareness and perception.

When January first entered the story, Wilson (Katie's husband) is summoned to pick up January from a nearby airport. January began retelling her brother-in-law her own origin story and how she ended up where she was with him. That moment offers readers another interesting vignette pertaining to the placenta as metaphor and metaform. At the airport catching a connecting flight, January encountered a mysterious woman, named Pearl, and her newborn child. Being newly pregnant January's interest was piqued. January here is depicted as young, green, and naïve, and she quickly befriends this woman who eventually steals her rental car and her beloved dog. January begins explaining her case to her brother-in-law over breakfast. While Wilson is spearing his steak and eggs at a local Denny's, after the airport incident, January explains simply and softly, "she knew about placentas." As January recounts her dialogue with the woman in said airport:

"Well January, Jan. Expect that life as you know it will soon end."

January didn't know what to say. "Forever." The woman smiled. Her name was Sophie. She was forty-two—older than January first thought—and had given birth to her daughter in her living room, in a plastic swimming pool. She was in labor for twenty-two hours. Water leaked into the apartment below and she was almost evicted, but it was worth it. She warned January that no matter what, she should not have her baby in a hospital.

"Why?" The coffee was bitter and sweet on January's tongue. The dog barked in its crate behind her.

"They won't give you the placenta." Sophie smirked. "It goes to pathology, like it's something dangerous, which I guess, to 'the man' it is."

"You mean the afterbirth?" January vaguely remembered her babysitter's cat eating a bloody hunk of something after having kittens. "Why would you want it?" "You eat it." Sophie acted like it was the most natural thing in the world. "You slice it up and cook it in a stroganoff. Or you can freeze dry it and stir it into shakes. It's exactly what the woman needs, nutrient-wise, after giving birth. It just seems weird because we've gotten so far away from the natural world." She sighed, resting her cheek on the baby's head. "Sometimes I think we are so co-opted, we're barely alive." (118)

In order to deconstruct such images from a feminist, psychoanalytic perspective, the cat-mother eating her own placenta after giving birth could be seen as a silent way to explain an almost unwanted pregnancy (155). This sealed-off memory of Jan's is protected and otherworldly, as she ponders her feline feminine power shortly after this recollection.

January, upon telling her story to Wilson, feels guilty, embarrassed, and ashamed for being taken advantage of so easily, especially by a person who seemed to be a fellow feminist. She then attempts to justify and explain away her most recent sin:

"But she was nice." January was like her sister in that she never conceded a point. It was so obnoxious it was charming. Her hair stood up in happy peaks, and her green eyes, narrow like Katie's, were bright.

"She knew about all sorts of things," she continued. "Stuff I'm interested in: having babies, the placenta, feeling like you're not a part of the world, like you're some sort of alien, and the thing is, it's not your fault, it's the world's fault..." January trailed off. "Anyway, that's what she said."

Wilson was silent. *It's not your fault, it's the world's fault.* He felt that often, but according to the program, that was wrong, it was only stinkin' thinkin' and would lead you back to just one place: the bottle.

"Wait, he said, sitting up. "The placenta? Why on earth would you be interested in *placentas* of all things?"

"Oh yeah, I'm pregnant," January mumbled, intrigued by her hash browns. (132)

It is significant to note how the book is written structurally. Each chapter is written from another character's perspective and it jumps back and forth in time. It is equally important that as readers, we first meet Jan through her dialogue with another woman, at an airport travelling to meet her sister, soon after learning that she is with child. However, we only hear her complete retelling and dialogical account of her narrative, as she speaks her truth aloud to her brother-in-law, Wilson. When Wilson drives January home to her sister Katie, more images of the placenta and the feminine abound:

"Happy?" She [Katie] turned to January, sitting by her side on the carpet, still in her pajamas, a creamy pink blanket wrapped around her shoulders. January nodded, pulled the blanket tighter. Her ankles stuck out of her too-short pants. If Katie squinted, the begonias looked like placentas, ripe and reddish-pink, blossoming all over her sister's skinny legs. For a moment, her heart filled with happiness. Another baby was on its way. And who was it, this little girl—for she was sure it was a girl—soon to plop herself into her crazy sister's life. (163)

Katie goes into her own dream state prompted and sponsored by the juxtaposition of the two sisters once again conjoined. Having been separated and now reunited, the two begin meditating on the possibilities of placentas:

Katie had often imagined giving birth at home. Pregnant with her own children, she'd lie in bed at night, picturing it as an underwater sort of experience, the air in her bedroom thick with silence, vibrating slightly with each contraction as moonlight poured through the windows onto the bone-white island of her belly, onto Wilson's strong hands, waiting to catch the new child. Then it would be time, and the baby would come, rushing from her in a rush of waters, rushing to Wilson who would place it on her belly, a briny, washed-up creature, it's sea-kissed face surprised and asleep, as she gathered it into her arms and up to her breast, awash herself on a tide of mother love. They'd nurse and sleep and sleep and nurse, getting to know each other, alone together in the seclusion of her room, lost in the twilight world of *after birth,* the moon rising and the moon falling, the baby warm and dry, its hair still caked with blood, its creases still waxy and white from the womb … Half here, half not—this was what she fantasized in a good mood. The other side of the coin was less pretty: She is in labor in her bedroom. It's a mess and she can't get her mind off the fact that she'd cleaned it just that morning and already it is trashed. Underoos and socks thrown everywhere, the bed covered with wet towels, graham cracker crumbs on the sheets, books—an explosion of picture books—making it hard to walk without slipping. And it's not the heart of the night, it's a busy bright Saturday afternoon, and through the wall the neighbor guy's stereo is blasting, annoying rap music, vibrating and thumping around in her room, vibrating and thumping around in her already too finely tuned body. (169-170)

In her daydreams, Katie illustrates both the positive and negative ways in which the birth can go. Creatively, Knutsen uses Katie as the protagonist in order to illustrate how an individual's thoughts, feelings, and constructed mythologies overlap with strong ties and parallels to the universal unconscious, the shadow selves each individual may experience.

Knutsen continues discussing images of the afterbirth and the plenitudes and platitudes of family life. She particularly ponders the relationship between mother and child through the budding friendship and dialogue between Lucy and January:

Calm down. Lucy grabbed her Big Gulp off the curb. It's

just the northern lights. Who cares? If you were from here, you'd know.

"I think Steven is cheating." She flopped her leg on top of January's. "Do *you* think Steven is cheating?"

"What do you mean?" January sensed a trap.

"Is your sister in love with Steven?" Lucy rested her hand on January's bare thigh, fingers poised to pinch. She was skinny in her T-shirt. Her hair was stringy, and she looked miserable, despite her night in rock n' roll heaven. Or maybe because of it.

"Let me put it this way." Lucy wiped her nose. "Is your sister screwing my fiancé?"

"No. God, no." January closed her eyes, bracing herself for the pinch. But it didn't come. When she looked up, Lucy was smiling—content, like a cat. She didn't say a word. January grabbed her hand, confused. Lucy's nails were dirty and chewed. (359)

With Lucy, Katie is in her consciousness as her arch nemesis, and Lucy herself resembles the cat that ate the placenta in their childhood. Lucy is a devouring image of the feminine, the feline, dirty and animalistic. This is one of January's last interactions with another woman, even another human person, in the story. She strikes out on her own, running away from her sister, her friend, and her son.

The network of leitmotifs that vary from person to person in the novel also seek to connect them through, once again, a primordial, shared, collective unconscious, the "dark mask," as if each character can inhabit the other's spectres or shadow selves. It is not that the deep symbolism of the placenta or other such prominent metaphors lead nowhere; instead, they lead everywhere, to more personal (both shallow and deep) connections. The modulated descriptions of consciousness that each character experiences, though perilously modern in its dilemma (of autonomy versus connection, of personhood versus nature), are not written or constructed in a rarefied environment. They also are not overly precious, as if the reader has to play some sort of intellectual game with the writer to figure out the symbols' meanings.

Another passage, later in the novel, explains how January got away with her slippery "disappearance," both in her own consciousness and in how she physically disappeared and ran away from her family and everything else she left behind:

> It did feel good to be clean. Katie had even let January use her good shampoo, after agreeing to babysit for the night—if January pumped first.

> "Then if we run out of breast milk, he can have some formula. One little bottle isn't going to hurt."

> "Or you could nurse him," Wilson had joked.

> "The day I start nursing someone else's baby..." Katie shook her head.

> "*Please,* January thought. *Take over, set me free.*" (348)

Through the women's silent pleading, intimacy and connections are made. Associational clusters—pertaining to the moon, other women, afterbirths, water, heartbeats, and other subtle vibrations—can be detected through Knutsen's subtext. Here is a sort of *l'écriture féminine*, writing in "white ink" or "with our two lips speaking to each other." The concepts originate in the poststructural feminist literary tradition, including the work of Hélène Cixious, Luce Irigaray, and Julia Kristeva. They posit, in what has been called an essentialist way, that women are closer to language, to the realm of the symbolic,[1] because of their bodies, birth experiences and/or regenerative, life-giving potentiality. As Cixous posits, "There is always, within her at least a little of that good mother's milk. She writes in 'white ink' with 'white ink,' breast milk feeding the child" (881). The two lips refer to women conversing with one another and also a woman knowing herself, her body. These writers are trying to link up the cerebral with the material, which I think Knutsen's text also attempts. This is particularly done so, again, through the dialogue between two friends, Jan and Lucy:

He probably can't get enough, Lucy rolled to her side, her head resting on her arm [inviting, proximally her connection, communication, association with her friend January]. Her body was covered with the shadows of vines.

"You may not have enough milk. My sisters never nursed, they didn't want to ruin their boobs. Put him on formula and you'll be fine."

"Like you know anything about babies." January pulled off her stinky pajama top and threw it in the bushes. The nursing bra was hideous—beige and enormous—but she was too tired to care. A fat bumblebee hovered near her ankle, buzzing peacefully....

"You don't even like Abby. And she's not a baby." January flipped onto her stomach, letting the sun warm her back. The hot cement felt good against her cheek. She drifted off. "Anyway," she mumbled, "I'm supposed to hold him all the time. That's why I have the Snugli. That's why he sleeps with me. It's attachment parenting. Katie says—"

Lucy looked aghast. "Jan, you can't let him sleep with you. You'll roll over and suffocate him."

"No. It makes him secure...." (346)

Many of the characters in Knutsen's text have vivid fantasy lives. They have daydreams and nightmares about getting away, being set free, and about family life in general. These fantasies compress, combine, confine, and abstract the characters' repressed and suppressed emotions into symbols (such as the placenta, the breast, the pen, the white milk/ink), as illustrated by their various perspectives and points of view. The characters' motives are hinted at by way of symbols, or implied. Different readers, depending on their own various subject positions, will attach and ascribe different and various meanings to these same symbols. We see motherhood as engulfment, as entrenchment, as literally being in the trenches. Though in our capitalist society, the male in the family is still the breadwinner. How far have we really gotten from Plath and Hughes's marriage, sexual encounters, and ways of living? Is the bed still the centre of sexual politics? Is it the academy? The workplace?

Although some feminist traditions reject the classifications of waves of feminisms as taxonomy, they are useful typifications of a politicized feminist agenda. If this is the fourth wave of feminism, it looks despairingly like the second. Be it Michigan or Court Green, the gables and shackles of motherhood vary with each engaging experience of it. Suicide is pondered. Addiction takes root. Wilson, a professor of English and gender studies, is writing a doctoral dissertation based on the work of a famous feminist foremother, Sylvia Plath. He begins to fear that he really "knows nothing about women." Readers are reminded here of "the feminine mystique," as Wilson lives in what he calls "the pink cave," whereas the women in Friedan's narrative are stuck ordering appliances and vacuuming on Valium, endlessly washing dishes, and changing diapers. Here it is Wilson who feels forced to take "buffers" of speed and benzodiazepines.

Consistently and constantly throughout the text, myths and metaphors of the feminine archetype are deployed and redeployed. These metaphors and symbols function to reinforce and under-score the importance of birth and rebirth—spiritual, professional, academic, and actual in various discursive formations. This is done chiefly through conversational analysis between characters. It is also achieved through a feminist narratology, which includes characters' personal, internal and interior monologues, physical descriptions of place and space: "The baby is born. Lovely [Katie's dog] bursts in, leaps about the room like a bucking bronco, sniffs disinterestedly at the new baby, then makes off with the placenta, the cord trailing behind him like the tentacles of seaweed he used to love dragging around on the beach in Oregon" (170). Through images of the placenta and themes of rebirth, the women in the text feel as if they have regained what is rightfully theirs.

The theory of mind, or consciousness, as presented by thinkers such as Heidegger, de Man, and Bachelard, and illustrated by the structure of the metaphors in the previous excerpts, show Katie's (the speaker here) cognitive processes as active, searching, not neutral and passive. Her mother-womb-water wish is like a searchlight under those same waters (or like a Woolfian lighthouse), unveiling some truth hidden beneath the well of wonder (the mother-child bond).

Even more telling is taking this analysis one step further in order to contextualize Knutsen's writing. Analysis is done not only in the realm of her critical feminist foremothers (Plath and Woolf), and of the process of baby making, but also of writing womankind in the English literary tradition itself (69). Knutsen is able to do this through her feminist narratology. In an interesting way, she inserts such theories into her text. An example of this occurs when Wilson is about to cheat on Katie with his colleague:

As he pulled away, Wilson thought again of Alice's exposé. Katie the psychoanalyst said that humans create their stories—the stories of their lives—subconsciously, choosing just the characters needed in order to learn and grow. Alice, it seemed, had created her story on a conscious level before it even happened. (213)

It is Wilson who proposes that his dissertation be a creative rendition of the lost journals of Sylvia Plath, he who works in the gender studies department at the university where he develops such classes as "media and gender." It is Wilson who becomes addicted to drugs after also having an affair with Alice Cherry, an adjunct professor and a part-time stripper with whom he works and with whom he seeks a journey of mutual empowerment (which of course, quickly turns to mutual disrespect). As Wilson (last name Lavender!) writes in the dissertation that he fears he will never complete: "Things begin to devolve."

By making the main characters academics, Knutsen purposefully invites her readers to critically analyze how people make sense of the world around them. In her work, we come to understand how characters think (through an intellectual process), how they experience the passage of time, how they see and perceive, how they dream, how they feel, and how the kinetic response is somewhat universal or primordial. This response can be invited into thought through the image of the placenta as myth and metaphor. As through the begonia as imagistic detail, readers observe and take part in a certain character's special subjectivity (how the book is divided into chapters by character rather than chronologically serialized). The primitive modalities through which such themes are explored are the abstraction, metamorphosis, transformation, compression, condensation, comparison of image, symbol, and metaphor, and how these modes trigger memories (both implicit and explicit) and ideas about the mysticism of birth. The book is written in a discontinuous manner, a form of retrospection, which is not consistent with chronological time. Instead, the "real time" that both the characters, and therefore reader, experience is really "psychological time." This measurement of time responds and passes for the reader/character in response to what they are experiencing, such feelings as excitement, boredom, lust, and love—familial, romantic, and platonic.

In order to remark on the style of Knutsen's writing, the biological connectivity to the placenta in specific, and the mode, experience, and method of motherhood in the general sense, readers can detect the placenta in multiple modes. For instance, literally, the placenta is the tissue and fluid in the body that is needed to create a new body, house a new consciousness. This is a requirement of the fluid sensations of the body, the link between past, present, and future, in terms of ensuring the survival of the human species. Readers are reminded of the Freudian triangle "mommy-daddy-me" "the penis-the pussy-the baby," even if it is only to radically question this heteronormative assumption. Two or more of the main characters of Knutsen's novel use mind-altering substances in the context of their experience of family life (the placenta being always at the centre, even taking the stage over the actual child to come). The sheer multiplicity—the bombardment, of stimuli and response, and cause and effect—happens in the moment of conception, childbirth, of word, of thought, of action, of deed. This microcosm of experience, then, leads to an enriching miniature world that the child will soon inhabit. A ponderous, wondrous world of sense-memory, stimulation, not bound to anything except the Lacanian notion of the mother as "real." The simple categories of how a character sees, thinks, acts, feels, and experiences time collapse. This is important in the realm of the symbolic, the realm of the parents, the individuated, the storytellers, the syntax, style, sentence, and diction. But this does not exist in the realm of the child or fetus whose whole world is the "real," the mother.

I argue that this pattern of tension and release is a key element to how the reader experiences the story. With the entry of Katie and January's babies, we infiltrate dreams of eyeless darkness but also dreams of splendour, with water births and caring midwives and doulas. It is a nightmarish vision (giving birth), but it is also bringing forth new life. In the mind of the mother, we glean this as a mystical or psychical state of being. The woman and child, once delivered, however painful or pleasant the state of delivery, whichever way the placenta follows, impose on the reader a state of supraconsciousness in a sense, a way to feel disembodied. The feeling is that the mother and child are one if even only for a fleeting moment, an instance in time, of being with time.

January's decision to abandon her child then leaves the reader in an anxious and fearful state, as she runs off to be with her former love lost—the 1980s hair metal band member Stevie Flame and her new friend Lucy. Katie, in the meantime, was cheating on her husband Wilson, with Lucy's soon-to-be husband, Steven. This complicates the Freudian triangle of mommy-daddy-me, and substitutes other surrogate parents.

A subliminal response is elicited in the reader (a click-murmur response) as soon as we hear the baby's heartbeat in an unfeeling doctor's office. The complex emotional reality and lived lives of the characters start ticking to that very drumbeat. Biological time triumphs over clock time from this point on. Characters' thoughts seem intuited by the reader, inferred through images, such as the heartbeat or the placenta, and then disentangled from the realm of the "real"—the mother's body at the point when she abandons her children.

Other metaphors exist here as well. For instance, when Jan is at the health clinic getting examined and hearing and experiencing that first ultrasound/sonogram, she is on a hard table in a stiff paper dress, juxtaposed against the soft roundness of the mother's stomach and her pillowing breasts. The tree—used for the paper gown and the examination table abstracted into things useful and at the disposal of humankind's purpose, an exploitation of nature—reminds the reader of sterility, of forced adaptation. A scrubbed, hard board table is a symbol of muscularity, youth, lumber, virtue, integrity, grained and knotted much like the inside of the mother's stomach as she prepares for a child she is ambivalent about having. The child's father used to bring Jan fruit—symbols of a lush life and prosperity. January sees herself, like the table, struck, suspended, the table's four legs paralleling Jan's two legs in stirrups. The table, with its personified and anthropomorphized legs, can symbolize humankind's feeble attempt to control and quantify nature and, by extension, womankind and childbirth.

Through the use of discontinuity, the reader is made aware of the fleeting nature and flow of life, birth, and thought. The novel radically questions the construct of a manufactured track to reality or wholeness. The two main characters are doctoral candidates, whereas the young mother and father are high school dropouts, and all are juxtaposed outside space and time. The emotional quality of these contrasts makes the reader feel as if there is something disingenuous in the hierarchy of education and pedagogy. While enriching, this hierarchy is not a part of the natural order of things, nor is it perhaps conducive to a mother's way of life.

ENDNOTE

1 In psychoanalytic language words including "symbolic" and "real" can also be capitalized to encapsulate Lacanian nuance.

WORKS CITED

Bachelard, Gaston. *The Poetics of Reverie: Childhood, Language, and the Cosmos*. Translated by David Russell, Beacon Press, 1971.
Cixous, Hélène. "The Laugh of the Medusa." *Signs,* vol. 1, no.

4, 1976, pp. 876-896.

De Man, Paul. *Blindness and Insight: Essays in the Rhetoric of Contemporary Criticism.* Routledge, 1983.

Freud, Sigmund. *Studies on Hysteria.* Edited and translated by James Strachey, Basic Books Inc, 1891.

Friedan, Betty. *The Feminine Mystique.* W.W. Norton, 1963.

Heidegger, Martin. *Being and Time.* Translated by John Macquerrie and Edward Robinson, Harper & Row, 1962.

Knutsen, Kimberly. *The Lost Journals of Sylvia Plath.* Northern Illinois University Press, Switchgrass Books, 2015.

Lacan, Jacques. *On Feminine Sexuality, the Limits of Love and Knowledge (Encore). The Seminar of Jacques Lacan.* Translated by Bruce Fink, vol. XX, book 20, WW Norton & Company, 1999.

Plath, Sylvia. *Ariel: The Restored Edition: A Facsimile of Plath's Manuscript, Reinstating Her Original Selection and Arrangement.* Harper Collins, 1999.

Woolf, Virginia. *To the Lighthouse.* Harcourt, Brace & Co, 1927.

17.
Snakes, Berries, and Bears

A Father's Placenta Story

CHRISTOPHER CORDONI

W E STROLLED ALONG THE DIRT ROAD, buckets in hand for the berries we picked along the way. Ripe blackberries were baking in the afternoon sun, filling the warm air with sweet, fruity perfume. All manner of flying insect droned, buzzed, hovered, and flitted among and around us. Shanti ran ahead, then stopped, peering straight down at the surface of the dusty road. She motioned pointedly with her finger at something, rotated toward us, and crossed her little arms high on her chest. We straggled toward her, engrossed in our labour as we continued to hunt for the fattest, juiciest fruit amid the prickly vines. On her face she wore an exaggerated scowl.

"Aww." she lamented. "It's dead." As we joined her, we saw that there, on the pale, dry, dusty road, lay another desiccated, flattened snake. Shanti crouched down into a squat directly over the sinuous form, and then reached toward the bushy roadside for a twig. She used this tool to hook one of the loops of the lifeless form, holding it upward as she observed it closely. She thrust it toward her older sister, Danaan. "It's so sad," she said.

"Let's bury it," suggested Danaan. She had accumulated a modest harvest of berries in her green plastic toy pail, which she eyed while reflecting thoughtfully. "Daddy, can I dump these into yours?" she asked, motioning toward the vessel I carried.

"Mais oui! But of course! Then I'll have even more to eat!"

"Not to eat, silly. To carry for me," she corrected, awaiting my agreement before upending her pail. With my grin, she proceeded to dump the plump, deep-purple berries that she had picked with care, and which had earned her a collection of minor scratches and burgundy-stained fingers along the way. Fruit fragrance wafted upward.

"Mmm. I think I have to eat some right now!" I said.

Bright smiling sisters took a generous mouthful each. Then Danaan extended the empty pail toward her sister. Shanti, deep in concentration, followed the movement of her own right hand carefully with her gaze as she balanced the suspended snake on its twig holder, proudly lowering it into the receptacle. "Did it!" she celebrated.

While Mother and Father continued to pick berries, the two sisters diverted their attention to a new task. One rescued snake in this berry bucket led to another, and another, and then another, as we made our way leisurely back to the cabin.

* * *

The plum tree was gnarled, riddled with wood-pecker holes, and stunted. It was a dwarf next to the towering red cedar overlooking the lake. It never produced much fruit, just enough for snacking as the days shortened and the evenings cooled with the waning of summer. We could see this year would be no different as the small developing, fruit hung sparsely from the tree's branches.

We crossed the small patch of browned grass encircling the trunk of the plum tree as we approached the little cabin, buckets laden, ready to divert our attention to preparing supper. The berries were destined to become jelly; we were unsure about the snakes. With two little ravenous children, we first had to get food on the table.

"Where will we bury the snakes?" queried Shanti later when we sat down to eat.

"Remember, we also have something else to bury," offered Mother.

We all understood this reference well. While not *the* reason for our visit to the cabin, the burial was to be a central activity. For three years, entombed in the back of the freezer, almost forgotten but ever present there in the dark, rested a human placenta. Once in a while Mother or Father would glimpse its plastic container when searching for something else more immediately required, like frozen strawberries or bread, perogies or peas. Each time, the same fleeting question remained unanswered: where will this material of birth and life, the placenta of our second child, find its peace, its final resting place?

* * *

The birth of our second child had been as joyous and traumatic as the first. On both occasions we envisioned a birth in the sanctuary of our own home. Although Danaan was birthed in our bedroom, we soon found ourselves in the hospital due to what appeared to be a breathing irregularity. With Shanti, birth at home was not realized. Things progressed slowly after Mother's waters broke, and we found ourselves the next day walking up and down Little Mountain, hoping gravity would help draw our little one downward. As evening came, labour became stronger, and continued into the wee hours, but as time passed, pain and pressure became unbearable. Without a midwife at home, Mother decided to move to the hospital, although we did not know the doctor who might be available to us there.

The rooms there were large, quiet, private. We relaxed for a few fleeting moments— dumbstruck to be there in that establishment, weary and disoriented, but relieved that it was tranquil, hoping that the birth would unfold on our terms. In no time at all, Mother, who had arrived fully dilated at the hospital, was pushing out this little person in the subdued light of the birthing theatre, surrounded by spectral instruments, alien implements, and two nurses. To my relief, it appeared that we were done, the unknown doctor arriving just at the moment of Shanti's crowning head. Our beautiful healthy baby girl had arrived peacefully into this world. Mother held her, as we gazed with love and awe, a new little girl in our lives—a moment of grace in the room.

But the process had not concluded. The cord—connecting Mother to daughter, daughter to Mother, and continuing to conduct necessities of life—was severed abruptly, the doctor acting with alarming haste, not heeding Mother's almost immediate request, "Don't cut the cord." He looked up in surprise at this urging. Our transient peace was now broken as he continued his interventions, coaxing the second birth, as I can only imagine now, very impatiently. No time in this place for the important second act of the placenta's birth.

The doctor climbed up on the gurney, standing over my partner who lay below on her back, clutching our child, placing his right foot on the inside of her left thigh, leaning back, applying his weight to the cord as if he were trying to drag a reluctant beast from its corral. At least that's the twisted image I conjure when I try to recall that early morning when Shanti was born. Did the doctor think his application of force was reasonable as he pulled on the cord, unrelentingly, seemingly without regard to the clear message communicated by Mother's body, by this organ, this placenta?

I'm not ready, it resisted. *I need time to separate as I must, to release this grasp, this bond as intimate as any connection can be*, it pleaded. *I am as much a part of this mother as she is of me, as we have grown together for nine months, as we have become one in this interconnected bundle of tissue and blood. As determined as you are to rip me out, I wish not to relinquish my rootedness from this place. Not yet. I know my job is almost done*, it reasoned. *Not quite yet.*

But this time was not allowed. The placenta gave way, not on its own accord, but to make peace, the doctor falling backward with its release, sprawling across the floor triumphant, glistening cord and organ flailing in his hands. I know this image is only another confabulation, but it's there rooted in my memory.

Our little baby was quickly taken from Mother's arms, brought to a tray far across the room in nurses' hands before either of us could emerge from our shared stupor and intervene. And so followed the blood, Mother's blood, as it flowed, weeping from the wound created by unknowing hands. This haemorrhage resulted in the loss of much blood from Mother's body, a body already exhausted from its act of life giving. Yet to our surprise, after intervention controlled this loss of blood, we were soon on our way home with our baby—and our placenta.

Mother was very weak, remaining bed ridden for a month, suckling and cuddling our baby, eating and sleeping in a small but intimate space. She was served freshly juiced beets in bed, fed leafy green vegetables, given "liquid iron" and even meat, meat for a vegetarian desperate to see herself restored. Her restoration was also supported by consumption of part of the placenta over several days, cut into small pieces, fried. Still retaining the necessities for life, it nourished again after its primary life-giving function was complete. The umbilical cord was left to dry in a spiral shape, and the rest, the bulk of this rich flesh, found its way into the back of our freezer.

* * *

Years passed, including a move from one apartment to another, and a faithful conveyance of the white plastic bucket from freezer to freezer. Again, it was placed into a back corner, plastered around with assorted frozen foodstuffs. We couldn't quite see this white plastic bucket unless we intended to, which was rare. More commonly it appeared accidentally in our quest for something else, and there and then we were forced to pause for a moment. This reminder, this placenta in the back of the freezer, the placenta that wouldn't let go, that refused to relent, continued to endure. Now it was affixed to the back corner of its cubicle, having forged bonds in frost and ice, connected again to its surroundings. But it begged for a more honourable fate.

At times it felt as of Shanti's placenta would remain a permanent part of our icebox, until inspiration struck late that summer. We lived in an apartment in the city and had no piece of land, no place to call our own, nowhere to inter this sacred piece of flesh. But up the coast, my parents kept a little cabin on a little lake, a patch of ground that would receive with dignity this stuff of life. In turn, finally, its matter would be liberated, free to infuse the soil, to spread its web infinitely beyond.

Out from the back of the freezer we pried the placenta and placed it carefully into our tiny cooler, beside some milk, eggs and cheese. No one had a clear idea exactly where the placenta would finally be put to rest, but there was a forest of trees and a patch of inhabited land in waiting.

* * *

"What about the plum tree? I'd like to bury the placenta there. That tree certainly needs some help," suggested Mother.

"What about the snakes?" chimed the two girls.

"And the snakes." It was agreed.

After finishing the supper dishes, I retrieved a shovel from the tool shed and proceeded to the tree. The girls brought their bucket of dead, mummified snakes, Mother the bucket of thawed, glistening placenta. Both Shanti and Danaan took turns trying to pierce the rocky earth, but it gave way only very reluctantly.

"No wonder this tree is having such a hard time," I thought aloud. "There's hardly any soil."

With some time and effort, we excavated a modest hole near the base of the plum tree, past a thick network of assorted roots. A small mound of jagged little rocks dusted with red soil lay piled beside us. Words were spoken, acknowledging the beauty of the snakes and their sad end, honouring life, death, life giving, and recognizing how Shanti and her mother were once connected intimately inside by this placenta. Both buckets were upended gently, conjoining a tangled mass of reptile, mammal, scaly skin, moist flesh, and tree roots within the cavity. You're not alone. Each in turn helped cover the contents with dirt and rocks. You're not alone.

We knew this accumulation of organic matter would nourish the tree in the weeks and months to come, but we also realized it may nourish a scavenging mammal that very night or soon thereafter. Racoons were common in the area, as were bears, both of which were normally kept at bay by a neighbouring dog. All three might be happy to feast on what lay at the bottom of the hole we had just filled. So on top of the disturbed area, we placed a large rock, large enough to flummox a racoon or dog, perhaps not secure enough to ward off a bear but as good as we could manage.

* * *

We continued to visit the cabin as often as we could. Summer turned to fall, to winter, to spring. Greens of all shades and hues exploded out of every corner of the landscape. Insects came to life as the sun's energy intensified, and swallows swarmed over the lake, engulfing mouthfuls of these newly-birthed creatures. We imagined that the plum tree's blossoms were more profuse than ever before.

This was the time for huckleberries, which we ate greedily, handfuls to mouthfuls, and cherished as the first bounty of the season, nature's gift after a grey winter. Sometimes we had the patience to try to fill little buckets, which invariably made their way back to the cabin containing only a meagre harvest. But we were contented having sated ourselves earlier. Those that escaped consumption until the morning were mixed into pancake batter.

"The plum tree looks happy," commented Shanti at breakfast. "I think we will have LOTS of plums to eat! When will they be ready?"

We had to be patient awaiting the plums; they would be the last to ripen in late summer, but we made certain to return to harvest them. It took until after school had resumed in early September to make the trip, and we were all curious to see what would await us at the lake. We arrived at the cabin at dusk to an astonishing scene. On the ground beneath the tree lay one of the tree's major branches, torn, shredded from its joint on the main tree trunk. On the trunk of the damaged tree were four claw marks deeply etched, running vertically two feet long. The downed branch had been ravaged, displaying the same etchings and bearing not a single plum. All had been eaten by a bear, a bear most certainly happy to fatten itself on sweet, ripe fruit.

But all was not lost. Shanti had been correct in her prediction. There was a bumper crop of plums; picking those that remained suspended from vibrant branches still provided more than we had ever picked before, enough to bring home and to eat fresh, to dry and to make jam, to share with family and friends, enough. Everyone who ate them commented on the rich, sweet succulent nature of our home-made plums.

About the Contributors

Alison Bastien has a degree in anthropology. She practised as a homebirth midwife for fifteen years in Mexico. For over twenty-five years, she has been a childbirth educator, herbal healing consultant, and teacher of midwifery and plant spirit medicine. Her hobbies include writing and quilting. Website: www.lavictoriana.com

Judy E. Battaglia is a clinical professor of communication studies at Loyola Marymount University in Los Angeles, California, USA, where she teaches classes in rhetorical methods, gender, theatre, and a class she created and developed called "For The Love of the Game: Gender, Sport and Communication."

Valerie Borek (aka The Momma, Esq.) is a mother, once-attorney, activist and author, placentophile, and founder of the Birth Rights Bar Association. She is on a mission to empower others, especially in medical rights and privacy. Valerie is a homebirth mom who chose to ingest placenta-raw and encapsulated.

Emily Burns is member of the Religion and Society Research Centre. Dr. Burns completed her PhD in the school of social sciences and psychology at Western Sydney University, Australia. Her research areas include the social and spiritual practices of childbearing women. She has published scholarly articles on the Blessingway ceremony, placenta rituals, and the meaning of home space for home-birthing women.

Janet Chawla is an activist, researcher, scholar, and founder-director of the NGO, MATRIKA. Her current involvement is with qualitative research of the Jeeva Project—gathering data from families, dais, and other providers in four remote areas of India. Ms. Chawla has lectured on Indigenous concepts of the body and birth nationally and internationally as well as written books, produced a play, and made a film called *Born at Home.*

Christopher Cordoni is a father and youth counsellor. He believes that human health depends upon intimate organic connections with the natural world, its cycles and rhythms, its matter, and its primal lessons. Our passage through time and space need only be mediated by our senses, our natural, life-giving wisdom, our love of self, of other, and of the material that has given us life.

Alys Einion is a senior lecturer in midwifery, programme leader for the Innovative HE Certificate in Maternity Care, lifelong feminist, writer, blogger, mother, and midwife. Her research interests include midwifery education; feminism and reproduction; motherhood; lesbian and queer families; women's life writing and narratives; and narrative construction. She is also a novelist, an avid and unashamed bibliophile, and an advocate for LGBT+ rights within the workplace.

Amyel Garnaoui, born in 1969 in Rome, Italy, is an art historian, a midwife, and a mother of three children.

Marie-Dominique Garnier is a professor of gender studies at the University of Paris-8 France. Marie-Dominique has co-directed two volumes on the works of Hélène Cixous— *Cixous sous X* (2010) and *Cixous Party/Partie de Cixous* (2014). Her latest book titled *Alphagenre* (2016) addresses graphically gendered regimes in contemporary discourse. She is also a translator of Madeline Gins's *Helen Keller Or Arakawa*, to be published in 2017.

Amanda Greavette lives and works in Ontario, Canada. She is busy raising five beautiful children, painting and serving her community. Amanda is a La Leche League leader and a member of "Friends of Muskoka Midwives," one of the few midwifery advocacy consumer groups in Ontario. She studied at the Ontario College of Art and Design and has exhibited in many solo and group shows.

Nané Jordan, PhD, is a scholar-artist and mother of two teenage daughters, with a working background in pre-regulation Canadian midwifery and postpartum doula care. Nané currently works as a sessional lecturer in art education at the University of British Columbia, as a family enhancement worker with Xyolhemeylh, and recently held a SSHRC postdoctoral fellowship in the Centre for Women's and Gender Studies at the University if Paris 8, France. Nané's love of placentas continues through her birth work, art, and writing, as does her interdisciplinary research into mothering, midwifery, birth, ecofeminist arts, women's spirituality, and well-being. Nané lives in Vancouver with her husband and daughters, where she admires the roots of both placentas and trees.

Nicole Link-Troen operates Richmond Placenta Encapsulation, providing safe, professional encapsulation services to women seeking to consume their placentas for the postpartum benefits. Since starting in 2010, she has handled, studied, and admired over 250 placentas, including 15 sets of "twincenta." With the support of her husband, tribe of friends, and her fantastic clients, she is raising her two young children and her business.

Barbara Alice Mann, PhD, is professor of humanities in the Honors College, University of Toledo. Author of thirteen books and over two hundred articles and chapters, she recently published *Spirits of Blood, Spirits of Breath* (2016) and the *Matriarchal Studies Bibliography* (2015), both with Oxford University Press.

Catherine Moeller is a Toronto-based artist who pursued her love of photography at Conestoga College in Kitchener, Ontario, and psychology at York University. She worked as a Toronto freelance photographer and documented her travels around the world. While working as a limo driver, after a motor vehicle accident, she completed a large series of drawings as a way to deal with her chronic pain. She has shown her photography, photo collages, drawings, sculptures and paintings in various galleries in Toronto and has recently completed work on a graphic novel about grief and motherhood.

Jonelle Myers is a practising sociologist in San Diego, California. She is currently an adjunct professor with the San Diego Community College District and a contract compliance manager with Father Joe's Villages, San Diego's largest homeless services provider. Jonelle is a member of the San Diego County Breastfeeding Coalition and an active participant in the local breastfeeding community. Jonelle is a mother, wife, sister, daughter, and student of the world.

Molly Remer is an ordained priestess who holds MSW, M.Div, and D.Min degrees. She wrote a dissertation about contemporary priestessing in the U.S. Molly and her husband Mark co-create original birth art jewelry, goddess sculptures, pendants, and ceremony kits at brigidsgrove.com. Molly has maintained her Talk Birth blog, http://talkbirth.me, since 2007, and currently writes about thealogy, nature, practical priestessing, ritual, ceremony, and the goddess. She is the author of *Womanrunes, Earthprayer,* and the *Red Tent Resource Kit.*

Jodi Selander began working with placentas in 2006 and launched placentabenefits.info that year. She created the Placenta Encapsulation Specialist Training Course in 2007, and now has specialists providing placenta encapsulation services worldwide. She is the author of *The Postpartum Survival Guide.* Jodi's artistic placenta portraits can be seen at placentalove.com.

Farah M. Shroff, is the principal of Shroff Consulting, a public health, education, and social issues consulting company, which focuses on research, writing, facilitation, and more. Dr. Shroff also works in the Department of Family Practice and the School of Population and Public Health in the University of British Columbia Faculty of Medicine.

Amy Stenzel practised as a DONA certified doula and is an International Placenta and Postpartum Association (IPPA) certified placenta specialist. She recently published an article in the autumn 2015 issue of *Midwifery Today* on the topic of placentophagy. She completed her BA in gender, women's, and sexuality studies at Appalachian State University in Boone, North Carolina.

Polly Wood, MFA Creative Inquiry, MA Women's Spirituality, is a multidisciplinary artist, performer, and independent scholar whose work is devoted to the preservation of the Sacred Feminine. Her research into women's cross-cultural rites-of-passage, menstrual consciousness, global economics, and the Sacred Feminine are creatively expressed through her music, dance, performance ritual, visual art, and writing. A birth worker for nearly twenty years, Polly currently serves women as a PBi Placenta Encapsulation Specialist.